THE SCENTED VEIL

THE SCENTED VEIL

Using Scent to Awaken the Soul

Carly Wall

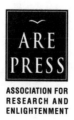

ARE
PRESS

ASSOCIATION FOR
RESEARCH AND
ENLIGHTENMENT

A.R.E. Press • Virginia Beach • Virginia

A.R.E. Press
215 67th Street
Virginia Beach, VA 23451-2061

Wall, Carly, 1960-
    The scented veil : using scent to awaken the soul / by Carly
Wall.
        p.   cm.
    ISBN 0-87604-442-9
    1. Essences and essential oils—Miscellanea. 2. Spiritual
life—Miscellanea. 3. Cayce, Edgar, 1877-1945. Edgar Cayce
readings. I. Title.
BF1442.E77 W35   2002
133'.254771—dc21

                                    2002005032

Cover design by Lightbourne

This book is lovingly dedicated to

My nephew Mike, who took me by the hand and showed me the world of computers. I couldn't have done it without you.

My co-workers at Lane Library, who pushed me on.

My mother, who introduced me to the A.R.E. as a child.

And everyone else in my life—you all have had a hand in shaping my work, and I am grateful and blessed.

Contents

Part 1: Ancient Powers Rediscovered

Part 2: Psychic Development

Author's Note

Essential oils are a scented, water-like fluid containing phytochemicals made by plants. These oils are highly concentrated and should be used with caution. Use sparingly and only as directed, especially the scents discussed here, since they do have effects on the mind. The frail or elderly, children, and pregnant women also should use care in applying the diluted essential oils to the body.

Part 1

Ancient Powers
Rediscovered

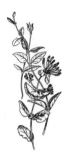

1

Harnessing Universal Energy

IN THE EARLY '70s, you would have found me at the community center, discovering Transcendental Meditation®. I tried to find my mantra, like everyone else, but meditation seemed so difficult. Next, I went on to yoga and learned the special breathing techniques. No one could tear me away from the television when my yoga show came on at 3:30 every afternoon. It made me feel so good. I became fit and slim—and it was very relaxing. But I still hadn't found what I was looking for, so I took some Zen meditation training. It was held above a shop that sold Native American-style merchandise. We climbed the narrow stairs to get to the darkened room where our teacher showed us how to twist ourselves into pretzel shapes and quiet our minds. But try quieting your mind when your legs are falling asleep and your back feels like it's holding up the Empire State Building. More than once, the teacher made me start over again, forcing me to face the wall. I think she was glad when I dropped out of class. Next it was on to Feldenkrais® class, where body movement is a form of meditation. I moved all over the place. I really enjoyed that class.

I've been to monasteries, taken dream retreats, and read all kinds of books—and all of it has been in search of one thing: to experience the power of altered states, to find enlightenment, to find my inner world.

All of us are searching for enlightenment, whether we are aware of it or not. Millions of books are sold each year on the subject. Did I ever find it? Yes, but it was a long and arduous journey. I can tell you what I learned along the way to make the journey easier. That's what this book is all about. Eventually, I found a meditation that has been good for me for more than four years. And I found out some other things too. When we are in search of enlightenment, we learn we are made up of not only a physical body, but also a psychic or inner self. And it isn't a new idea.

Every culture from the beginning of time has had its "secret societies" who have claimed to have found the answer to the way of altered states as keys to enlightenment. The mystics and philosophers of old often kept secret the methods they taught students to reach enlightened states, which they claimed were a pathway to unlimited power. If you were to study each of these paths to power, you would come away with one conclusion: that the universe teems with an energy, a power that is creative and is there for anyone to use to one's advantage—if one knows how.

For many years, this hidden or occult knowledge was suppressed, but just in the last few decades, it has become more accepted, and there has been an explosion of books, television shows, and articles about such knowledge. People have come forward to share their stories or amazing abilities. Genuine psychics are gaining new respect, and there are even psychics who help the police to solve murders. Since the early 1960s, when achieving altered states through whatever means was "in," we have learned a great deal about the potential of the human mind, a potential that only now has begun to be rediscovered after being nearly obliterated unknowingly by the Western mind view. Starhawk, a well-known writer and teacher of magic, ritual, and psychic development, has made it quite clear that all human beings have the potential to go into altered states. She talks about states that help one to obtain information unavailable in normal conscious states—states of ecstasy and states that can help one to create new realities where they can have whatever it is they want out of life. Swami Muktanada has been said to be capable of awakening spirituality in people with a mere glance or touch, causing great releases of a tremendous force called the *kundalini* energy. Joseph Campbell, author and well-known authority on myth and culture, often came across the subject of kundalini awakening in his researches. The phenomenon is apparently well known to mystics of India and can be awakened with complicated rituals. Such rituals help in spiritual unfoldment and purify or activate the body's energy centers or *chakras.* Actually, if you study any of the ancient cultures, you can see amazing parallels among civilizations in their beliefs about and practice of altered states. You can find similarities associated with aboriginal healing ceremonies and shamanic traditions of each race, from Native American to ancient Egypt.

Altered states are our link to our spirit core. I am convinced that it is a normal ability to be able to contact this spirit self and that we have merely moved away from it in our quest to overcome our physical world. We are made to be able to go into altered states, and there are many different tools we can use that can aid us in getting into these states. Some use meditation, some drumming, some crystals or candles. Whatever method we use, it is just our way of getting there. And what rewards when we do get there! This energy can be used, if used correctly, to grant us our fondest wishes, create wealth, find our true love, or locate our own fountain of youth. But so far, attaining mastery of altered states and of this energy has been perceived as a very difficult task. Until now.

I believe I have found a secret the ancient societies used to help speed the process and enhance it. From the time I was a little girl, scent has been an important part of my life, ranking right up there with my psychic and paranormal interests. My first garden was a scent garden, and I never bought canned air fresheners, but used only my homemade concoctions and potpourris. Eventually, from my interest in herbs was born a passion for aromatherapy. This love has turned into a career choice, and I am continually upgrading my education in that field. But here is where it gets interesting. Although I have often come across references to incense being used in religious ceremonies, I never really paid that much attention until I began to notice a pattern of particularly good meditation results that happened only when I used scent during my sessions. It suddenly dawned on me that, when I used scent, and especially certain types of scent, I got results. *Big* results. I believe that scent is one of the fastest, easiest, and most effective ways (when combined with other methods or tools) to alter awareness and gain access to unlimited power. In this book, you will discover how to awaken, develop, and use these powers through the use of various scents, along with other enhancing tools that work especially well together. Let's start by learning all about this mysterious power.

ALL ABOUT ENERGY

In chemistry class, I learned that energy can never be destroyed, only transformed. That was a mind-blowing concept for me, coming as it did from my eighty-year-old, wizened chemistry teacher. She always had a secretive grin on her face that made me feel that she knew something she wasn't going to share with the rest of us. Perhaps it was just that she really understood that concept. If energy can't be destroyed, I reasoned, then we can never die! Life is a continuous circle of transformation. From there, my lifelong researches began.

THE LUNAR CONNECTION

Our bodies, just like the planets, stars, moon, rocks, animals, and insects, all follow the ebb and flow of some energy that pulses through the universe. It is a continuous and creative energy, all-powerful. Ancient man was well aware of this energy. The early religions of Sun and Moon worship attested to the fascination these first worshippers had with the workings of the various heavenly bodies and how they affected life on the earth. This outside influence was found to affect people in individual ways (and so astrology was born, and we use it even today to predict events).

We again find mention of mysterious energy forces in ancient Chinese beliefs, a force called *chi*. Chi was believed to be a life energy that flowed throughout the universe, containing both yin (positive or male energy) and yang (negative or female energy) and often symbolized as the double-headed snake. This division of energy into male and female was quite common in other cultures as well. There are even references that the sun was believed to contain male or positive energy while the moon contained a negative or female energy.

Eventually, I came to believe that these ancient cultures knew far more about this energy than we do today. I don't know much about batteries, but I do know that the connections have either a positive or a negative charge (and I don't jump car batteries with jumper cables because I'm afraid I'll get them wrong and blow something up). Everything seems connected and governed by this energy. In fact, each of the tiny cells in our bodies are like little universes unto themselves. And today, yogis, acupuncturists, and healers all agree that the human body is a network of energy channels covering the whole physique. I have experimented with this energy and found it exists in animals, insects, and even plants.

Often, the Earth has been referred to as a living body, which makes sense in the whole scheme of things—everything is alive with a wonderful and powerful energy flow. Some people have been experimenting with this energy that seems to flow through the Earth. There are several books on the subject, and each of them confirms the belief that universal energy flows through all things everywhere. Could it really be true? Let's put it to the test to see.

The ancients took care to leave behind bits and pieces to the puzzle, so that we who came after could put the pieces back together. Wonderful testaments to their beliefs survive to this day. These religious sites are deemed very powerful or sacred. The Great Pyramid and Sphinx in Egypt are merely two examples. There are other pyramidal structures around the world, great stone megaliths, cave drawings, and earthen mounds as well.

Perhaps the ancients knew such powerful information could not be left to just anyone, and that, sometime in the future, people would rediscover such secrets when they were ready for them. Could our ancestors actually have harnessed the powerful energy that, today, we are only beginning to realize is there? Could it have become a dangerous weapon in the wrong hands and have been the seeds of destruction? We have myths about the lost civilizations of Atlantis and how Atlanteans harnessed a great energy that caused the island to sink. Many ancient cultures mysteriously vanished or ended. Think about it. In our time, we discovered nuclear energy and, ever since, have been struggling to come to terms with the fact that, with one push of a button, we can destroy the whole Earth as we know it now. It seems we have a pattern going here. Are we ready to again become empowered with this knowledge? I think the danger lies in not understanding clearly enough how powerful such knowledge is. Perhaps, since we have averted nuclear war so far, and, perhaps, since we are entering into the Aquarian Age, the age of understanding, it is time we understand the power of this knowledge in order to use it wisely.

A JOURNEY IN TIME

There are many interesting things about sacred sites. One is that they seem to all be astrologically aligned. However, it is the experimentation with dowsing that has created so much excitement of late. There is a belief among dowsers and some researchers that many of the stone circles and megalithic structures have geomagnetic peculiarities. For the book *Earth Magic,* (Pocket Books, 1978) author Francis Hitching clearly did extensive research on the subject of Earth forces and how man has had a connection to that subject since the beginning of history. Hitching told the story of Guy Underwood, a researcher who spent more than twenty years dowsing ancient sites such as Stonehenge and the Cerne Abbas Giant. Apparently, a great many of the power spots were found to be located above underground streams or even intersections of waterways. Underwood, said Hitching, believed he had identified a universally powerful "'earth force,' known instinctively to animals and plants and used from megalithic times onward by priesthoods to locate the communities' sacred centers . . . Instances from all over the world back up his findings."

Paul Devereux, author and director of the Dragon Project, a research project designed to study ancient stone structures, has, along with his volunteer researchers, documented amazing energy readings somewhat like ultrasound, at Rollright Stones, a megalithic site near Oxford, England. Geiger counters detected a higher count of radiation within the circle than outside it. This isn't surprising, given that sacred sites of Native Americans often sit atop uranium deposits. In France, the areas with the highest density of megaliths are often uranium-rich zones.

Dowsing is a way of detecting energy and has been used through the centuries as a way of finding water, although other items have been discovered using dowsing techniques, and it can be used in many different ways. Several dowsers have used this method on ancient stone sites and found that the energy currents swirl in corkscrew fashion around the stones. Nor should this be surprising, given that many of the power megaliths have been found to contain a large amount of quartz crystal, and we know that the molecular structure of quartz is also spiral.

The circle, which ancient humans were careful to include in some fashion in their monuments atop these energy gateways, has always been the symbol of eternity. The spiral (or corkscrew) is an ancient symbol of the progress of the human soul toward spirituality. As we spiral up toward eternity, we then move around the center and simultaneously outward. The spiral is a symbol of reincarnation, the way of the journey of souls. Spirals also hold the secret of life, which the ancients well knew. We know that the DNA molecule that transmits the genetic code is shaped like a double spiral or helix. Ancient man often used the symbol of snakes, and the symbol of healing and knowledge comes to us in the physician's emblem (caduceus) that depicts two snakes twined together, forming another double spiral.

As if that isn't clear enough, the ancient myths of India show that the Indian god Vishnu preserved cosmic order by coiling the serpent around the axis of the world, causing the forces of Good and Evil to pull the serpent in opposite directions. In Newgrange, Ireland, spiral carvings are found on stones leading to a tomb believed to be a temple to the sun; the spirals represented rebirth at winter solstice. The cave drawings of primitive man abound with drawings of snakes and coils. There is not one culture which hasn't depicted in some way a snake or spiral. In China, there is an ancient system of belief called *feng shui*. Feng shui is a system of energy flow, and emphasis is placed on how this flow affects humans— both positively, and negatively—in our awareness of earth energy and its flow through our homes and other surroundings. It has long been thought that proper energy flow could bring good luck to the family or persons who knew how to place objects so that the energy flow was at its best. The Chinese depict this energy flow with the symbol of dragons with coiled bodies.

We see spirals occurring in nature, too. There are spiral shapes of shells, the spiral of a spider's web, the spiral of water as it goes down the drain, and the spirals of storms as the winds whirl. Life is perpetuated by the double spiral, the yin and yang, the male and female energies combined. This double spiral is the basis of movement, the way to envision the great energy that flows through all matter.

THE OLD SNAKE

There are many places on the landscape dotted with so-called power spots. You won't have far to travel to find one of these sacred areas, either. Less than two hours from my home are several such places. The Miamisburg Mound is located near Dayton, Ohio, for example, and the Serpent Mound is located outside of Peebles, Ohio. These are shaped earthworks created by the Hopewell Indian culture. From about 500 B.C., mound building was at its zenith among Native Americans in the Midwest. These mounds come in a variety of shapes, including bears, birds, and human figures. But one of the most popular shapes had to be the snake.

On a cold and blustery day in October, I resolved to see the Serpent Mound for myself, so a friend and I set off on our adventure. We climbed the tower to take in the view and saw a giant earthen snake coiling over several acres at the site. We saw the spiral motion of the snake's body (the tail tightly coiled) and the triangular head of the snake that looked as if it were trying to swallow an egg (or circle?). The park was well-kept, and paved sidewalks followed the curve of the snake's body all around. Signs warned that visitors weren't to touch anything or walk outside the sidewalks. A sadness enveloped me. Although I knew that the thousands of visitors could destroy the site with tramping feet, it still seemed tragic that we flock to see such prehistoric sites only to come away not comprehending what it is we are seeing.

As such monuments go, it is not one of the largest, stretching merely a thousand feet long and six feet high. As we walked along the side of the snake to the head, we found it faced outward toward the edge of a cliff. The view encompassed the valley and surrounding hills. It was quite impressive. I even took a chance and sat along the edge of the circle. I felt nothing out of the way, but I have come across a few reports of others who have experienced strange occurrences. One man is reported to have stood upon the Serpent Mound and seen the strange sight of leaves gathering themselves together and walking toward him. He hurried to grab his camera from the car and found the moment was lost. There are other reports of incidents at other sacred sights too. At Stonehenge, several people have reported strange electrical shocks, visions, and other phenomena.

Disappointed that I hadn't been one of the lucky few, I walked on around to the other side. When I reached the coiled tail, it suddenly dawned on me that the mound, somewhat flattened at the top, would make a perfect walkway. The circle, with the depressed area in the middle, was the perfect arena. I felt certain these mounds had to have been ceremonial centers used to experience earth energy, but I also felt something was missing. Recently, I stumbled upon a newspaper account that made the missing piece clear, a piece that, for me, was the key to the secret of the mounds. The newspaper article reported that the site had been carefully surveyed several times, proving that the snake was carefully constructed with important astronomical alignments in mind, solar as well as lunar.

It is becoming increasingly clear to investigators that both the Hopewell culture and the historic Anasazi people of the American Southwest constructed sacred sites along astronomical alignments. Hopewellian structures in other areas such as the Great Circle in Newark and the Highbanks complex near Chillicothe, Ohio, all have astronomical alignments that previously were overlooked. The prehistoric Anasazi designed and built stone ceremonial chambers that had openings in alignment with the summer solstice. Some researchers now believe it was a calendar system used to tell the people when to plant and harvest crops. But what if the ancient people had something different in mind?

A line drawn from the center of the Serpent Mound's coiled tail to the center of the neck points to the North Star. A line drawn from the center of its neck through the center of the oval at the head (the egg or circle) aims toward a rise on the horizon where the sun sets on the summer solstice. And the three great eastward-pointing convolutions of the coiled serpent are in alignment with the summer solstice, autumnal equinox, and winter solstice sunrises. Why would these precise alignments be so important when planting and harvesting times can be calculated by watching for signs in nature that occur without having to go to all the trouble of building these monuments? There had to be another reason to calculate so perfectly. Instead, perhaps, these sites took advantage of a law of nature that helped ancient man understand and use a powerful force.

SWIRLING ENERGY

Sedona, Arizona, has become a magnet to spiritual seekers. It is being promoted as *the* place to go for experiencing earth's energy. According to Pete Sanders, author and president and founder of the Free Soul Psychic Education Program based in Sedona, Sedona's location is a concentration of *vortices*, or energy doorways. He says there are different types of energy patterns in the Sedona area, primarily "upflow" patterns and "inflow" patterns. The upflow vortex is expansive, touching oneness with the infinite; the inflow vortex turns the person inward to focus on old conflicts and past lives.

Thousands of years ago, the Sedona area was a meeting place for Native Americans from all across the Southwest. Experts concur that it was a great religious center. No one knows why it was abandoned a century before the Spanish entered Arizona, but its inhabitants left behind a legacy of stories that talked of spirals, snakes, and circles.

Symbols were often used by ancient priests and shamans to convey important truths. Symbols also helped to shield spiritual truths from those not ready to handle them. The Bible is one example of a story told in symbolic form. In Genesis, Adam and Eve in the Garden represent the male and female energies. Temptation comes in the form of a snake, which twines around the Tree of Knowledge of good and evil. The two ate of the fruit of this tree, misusing their power, and were banished from the Garden. Another example hails from ancient Egypt, where myths of twin snakes are plentiful. One was called the dragon, a bringer of good and light. The other serpent was of dark and evil.

The Egyptian story of Isis is particularly intriguing. Isis was weary of the world of men and yearned for the world of the gods (altered consciousness). She meditated in her heart, saying that she wanted to make of herself a goddess, like Ra, the Egyptian god of the Sun who had been ruler of Egypt and was given godly stature for his mastery of inner power. But Ra had many names, and the great name that gave him power over the other gods and men was known to no one but himself. So Isis planned another way to gain power. She gathered up Ra's spittle that had fallen upon the ground, kneaded it into earth and made a serpent of it. The sacred serpent stung Ra, and he became ill. Notice the words *meditate* and *serpent?* Notice also that such energy can be dangerous, for even Ra became ill from it. Isis took what little she knew about energy and used it against Ra.

The priests of Amen-Ra regularly held a ceremony that they believed helped to keep the world in check. They fashioned a serpent of many coils, made of wax. They called this the evil snake Apep, who fought to keep the sun from rising. In this ceremony, the snake was held in check so that the sun could always rise.

In China, the symbol of the dragon meant protection, good luck, rejuvenation of mankind, and immortality. The African Issapoo tribe on the island of Fernando Po regarded the cobra as a guardian deity, doing good or ill, bringing riches or disease and death. The skin of one of these reptiles was hung tail down from a branch of the highest tree in the public square in an annual ceremony. The Warramunga of central Australia believed in a mythic snake called Wollunqua, which lived in a pool. When they spoke of it among themselves, they called it by other names, for if it were called upon too often, they would lose control over the creature, and it would come up out of the water to eat them all up.

You will see how interesting these stories are when we delve more deeply into kundalini meditation in later chapters. For now, what emerges is a force, depicted as a double snake or serpent, that can bring great good in the form of healing, fertility, and eternal life, or, if misused, can rain down destruction, darkness, and death.

Clearly, these stories related to the energy force that flows through everything. But was this force harnessed and used in ancient times, and if so, how?

Francis Hitching talked about activated stones the ancients used as transmitters to absorb Earth energy. Hitching added, "For most people in the tribe, probably no special gifts were needed. Nowadays, such power as there is in the stones seems too unpredictable to be used in this way. Either people have lost the ability to absorb the power consistently, or the force has changed in character."

But suppose we are only seeing part of the picture. Suppose the force is still the same, unchanging. And also suppose that the power inherent can be controlled and harnessed consistently. And what if the answer is there right in front of us? What if we aren't "absorbing" the energy at all? What if our bodies, containing the energy, as we know all matter does, is part of the equation. What if we are supposed to tap into the energy, combine it with the Earth's energy, and so, enhance our ability to increase and direct it? What if the Earth's energy merely is a tool that helps awaken our own energy? These vortices of energy then, swirl not only outside ourselves, but within us, within the earth, and throughout the universe. Perhaps, in our rediscovery of forgotten knowledge, we, too, will be able to do many miraculous, wondrous things. Some people still experience strange occurrences at known power spots, so we know the power is still there. But just how did the ancients train themselves to work their magic?

We have only to explore the most ancient of our religious beliefs to find the answer. As we have seen in examples of the Judeo-Christian beliefs, the serpent is ever the symbol of good and evil. In one ancient manuscript written in Aramaic, the language of Jesus of Nazareth, we find that Jesus was trying to bring in New Age-type thought two millennia ago. References to a force within us in the form of a serpent, that can be used for our good, can be deciphered if we remember that symbolism was heavily used in His teachings. The Khabouris Manuscript of the Syriac New Testament, translated directly from its original Aramaic, gives us a truer version of what the authors actually meant, than is found in subsequent translations. The translation in John 3:13 originally read, "No man *rises* to heaven, except he who descends from heaven . . . and just as Moses *raised* the *serpent* in the wilderness, so is it necessary to *raise* the Son of man, so that all men who believe in Him will not be lost, but will have for themselves eternal life." And perhaps we get a feel for what the energy force is in this translation from John 4:23-24, " . . . worship the Father as *rukha* [emphasis added] and also as truth . . . Because God is rukha and those that worship Him as rukha and as complete truth are worshipping Him as they should." Now what exactly is rukha? In the glossary, the translators list this word as meaning *spirit, energy, wind, electricity. A quality of force* [Emphasis added].

THE MIRACLE OF KUNDALINI

In Hinduism, one of the major world religions and so ancient that it has no recorded history of its beginning and no founder attributed to it, there is also the tale of a snake. Hinduism reveres all life. Followers are expected to follow vegetarian diets; believe in one God, Brahman, the One that is All; and believe in reincarnation and karma. Within this religion is a doctrine of three paths of escape from the cycle of karma: duty, devotion to God, and knowledge sought through the practice of meditation and yoga. Hatha yoga, as this version is called, is the preparation of the body to be used as an instrument toward union with God. The true goal of a yogin (master of knowledge), was to talk to God through the use of meditation, which awakens the kundalini force. This force is described as a power that lies coiled like a snake at the base of the spine. The trick is to awaken this power and direct it upward, so that it flows through all seven spiritual centers or *chakras* to the highest spiritual center, the pituitary area between the eyes, also called the third eye.

Obviously, mastery of this energy means spiritual enlightenment. If one attains "enlightenment," one is revered by others in the group, clan, or tribe. Many other cultures seemed to have such a belief, or at least to have experimented with it, but used veiled language in referring to this dangerous knowledge. The Hopi passed on a tradition of teaching about energy centers in their mythic creation stories. The Kabbalists refer to the "seven gates in the soul of man." The early esoteric Christians used the code term "seven churches in Asia." The alchemists of medieval Europe spoke of seven metals or "planets." And the Rosicrucians taught about the "seven roses or inner stars."

It was obvious that these teachers, yogins, and high priests, wanted the mainstream of followers to believe that mastery of this power was difficult. Remember that this energy is both positive and negative and can be used for good and evil. Only those seekers who had proven their dedication, high ideals, and mastery of the body could safely be entrusted with the knowledge. This knowledge may have been lost because a few who weren't properly trained or motivated misused it. There is frequent mention in ancient stories of the laws of nature that tell us that those who misuse the force to bring death and destruction had, in every case, the negative energy rebound back upon them. In such a case, knowledge could indeed be lost.

Once one has developed the ability to move the kundalini energy through the energy centers, it is said that psychic powers become manifest. Ancient writings tell of acquiring the ability to know all, including the future and the past (precognition and retrocognition). Other abilities mentioned are knowing the thoughts of others (telepathy), the ability to go without food or drink, the ability to rejuvenate the body and live as long as wanted, the ability to levitate or become invisible at will, the ability to travel the astral planes, and the mastery of many other amazing abilities.

Edgar Cayce, called the sleeping prophet, gave psychic health and "life" readings in an altered state for thousands of searching souls during his lifetime. He had quite a bit to say on the subject of kundalini:

And if there will be gained that consciousness, there need not be ever the necessity of a physical organism aging . . .

Know then that the force in nature that is called electrical . . . is that same force ye worship as Creative or God in action!

Seeing this, feeling this, knowing this, ye will find that not only does the body become revivified, but by the creating in every atom of its being the knowledge of the activity of this Creative Force . . . spirit, mind, body . . .are renewed. 1299-1

PLUGGING INTO POWER

The upper three chakras are called our spiritual centers. These enable us to connect to the Universal Energy. In these upper chakras, the energy flow's function is blessing, embracing, and becoming. The lower four chakras, where it is believed our kundalini energy now resides because of our materialistic focus, are called the material or physical centers. When we focus most on physical pleasures, we can become trapped in these lower chakras. This downward flow also has a threefold function: creation, preservation, and destruction. Some believe the "fall" of man was really the downward flow of kundalini, as humans made the mistake of focusing too much on the physical. They were cast from Eden, so to speak, and only with sufficient knowledge, can they make their way back. The existence of such a way back is guaranteed, however, as we can see in Genesis 3:24: "So he drove out the man; and he placed at the east of the Garden of Eden Cherubims, and a flaming sword which turned every way, to keep the way of the tree of life." Matthew 7:7-8 promises that the way is available to all: "Ask and it will be given to you. Seek and you will find. Knock and the door will be opened for you. For everyone who asks receives and everyone who seeks finds; and to the one who knocks it will be opened."

The way back requires getting the energy flowing to

the higher centers once again. Basically, this involves visualization and rhythmic breathing so that the chakras, often represented as mystical whirling wheels (again, spirals), draw the vital force toward the top of the head.

As mentioned in the beginning of the chapter, there also are ways to increase and amplify this force. One is to connect to the Earth energy. We can easily tap into earth energies through the use of the crystal energy that spirals in quartz crystal or—and this is important—by using the vibratory qualities of particular scents. Matter is vibrating energy. Higher levels of vibration enhance Earth energy. That is why power spots often are linked to water; the water's vibration enhances the energy. And that's why rituals of cleansing and diet help—they elevate the vibratory qualities of the flesh, speeding results. Scent may provide an even faster way to raise these vibrations.

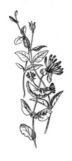

2

The Perfumed Temple

Talk not of temples, there is one
Built without hands, to mankind given;
Its lamps are the meridian sun
And all the stars of heaven
Its walls are the cerulean sky,
Its floor the earth so green and fair,
The dome its vast immensity,
All Nature worships there.
"The Temple of Nature"
                    —David Vedder

HOW IMPORTANT IS scent to us? Think about our obsession with "good" smells. Ads on television tell us we can banish all the "bad" body odors with this product or that. Certain laundry products can make our wash smell fresh and clean as a spring breeze. The latest perfume to come out tells us that this scent is sure to drive the opposite sex wild. Has it always been this way? Archeologists say yes. Research has proven that humans have had a long love affair with scented plants. They have been used as medicines, balms for the body and mind. They have also been used for pleasure. But there is another use that hasn't gotten much press, and that is their use in religious and magical rituals. Apparently, humans used scent first and foremost in religious ceremony. And I don't think this was an arbitrary choice. At some time far back in history, someone discovered that the use of scent could alter the mind. As experimentation and experience increased over the years, people found that some scents were more powerful than others, some could be used to elicit specific responses, and others were healing to the psyche or the physical body itself. At some time over the centuries, the importance of this finding was lost. Perhaps the meaning behind the rituals became lost in the routine of the actions themselves.

Take, for example, the Catholic Church, which uses incense to this day in its rituals. The most important scent used in incense has been frankincense, also called "holy smoke." From ancient times, it was regarded as a treasure and was traded as such. It has been said to be the highest of the mind-elevating scents and valued the same as gold. It even was recorded in the Bible as one of the gifts the three Wise Men chose for the baby Jesus. Yet, we are surprised in modern times that it has such power.

In 1981, scientists in Germany were called in to investigate a strange happening in a church. The altar boys were reported to be getting "high" on the smoke from the incense. During their investigations, the scientists found that the frankincense resin, when burned, produces a chemical called trahydrocannabinole, a psychoactive substance. The result is that this substance has the power to send the mind into another dimension of awareness.

Plants contain essential oils, chemical messengers the

plants use in a similar way to our bodies' use of hormones. A hormonal system for plants? Perhaps. But more
importantly, not only can the plant use these chemicals
for their survival—for killing bacteria and molds, attract-
ing pollinators, or repelling enemies—but the chemicals
also are useful to us. Often, the various scents have been
found to affect us profoundly.

THE THERAPY OF SCENT

Aromatherapy is the use of aromatic essential oils distilled or extracted from plants or trees. Usually, the
therapy consists of absorbing the material, which has
been diluted in a base oil, through the skin, either through
massage or by adding the essential oils to a bath. Another
method is inhalation. Ingestion (taken by mouth) is not
recommended for the average person and best left to
professionals, as these substances are highly concentrated
and sometimes dangerous. Modern aromatherapy got its
start from a French chemist, Rene-Maurice Gattefosse, in
1928, who did extensive research into essential oils and
their healing qualities. In his work, he was able to ob-
serve that the whole, pure essential oils were much more
effective than using only some of their components created in a lab. Another important player in the development of aromatherapy was Dr. Jean Valnet, who
successfully used aromatherapy treatments for both
physical and psychiatric complaints. The results of his
treatments were published in 1964 under the title,
Aromatherapie. Marguerite Maury keenly followed Valnet's
work, taking aromatherapy to the next stage. Her focus
was on the rejuvenating and beautifying effects of essential oils. Her research results were published in the famous work, *The Secret of Life and Youth,* which also came
out in 1964. She set up the first aromatherapy clinics in
Paris, Britain, and Switzerland. The European commu-

nity and the rest of the world now enjoy the benefits of aromatherapy, thanks to the hard work and persistence of these modern researchers.

Because of them, we know that pure essential oils, which are highly concentrated extracts from plants, flowers, resins, barks, roots, and seeds, can be very healing to the body, mind, and spirit. Some of these essential oils have the ability to penetrate cell walls and transport oxygen and nutrients, enhancing and building up the immune system. The chemical makeup of some of these volatile substances heals a variety of physical conditions, including skin problems, digestion, and infections. Aromatherapists have long known that using thyme or eucalyptus, for example, cuts short the effects of colds or flu by up to 50 percent because of their antibacterial and antiseptic qualities.

We also know that our sense of smell is very important to us from birth, and that, when we detect a scent, a specific portion of the brain is affected; namely, the limbic area, once called the "old brain," which is associated with mood, emotions, and memory. It has been shown that smells can be recalled with 65 percent accuracy after a year, while the recall of a picture is accurate at only 50 percent after just three months. Recent research has shown that fragrance has a positive effect on our alertness, and it is now being studied to improve job performance.

We are now becoming aware that essential oils also affect us in other ways, including our spiritual selves. Psychic Edgar Cayce, hinted at such exciting news in the latter part of the last century.

In reading 274-10, he stated:

For as has been indicated, and as may be or should be worked upon or classified by man, there is the ability to make odors that will respond, and do re-

spond, to certain individuals or groups; and many
hundreds *are* responding to odors that *produce* the
effect within their systems for activities that the psychoanalyst and the psychologist have long since discarded—much as they have the manner in which
the Creative Forces or God *may* manifest in an individual!

What meaneth they of old when saying: "This
hath ascended to the throne of grace as a sweet sav-
iour, a sweet incense before the Maker, the Creator,"
but that that within the individual is made aware of
that estate which he had before he entered into the
flesh and became contaminated by the forms of matter in such a manner? For odor is gas, and not of the
denser matter that makes for such activity in individuals' lives as to make for the degrading things.

What bringeth the varied odors into the experience of man? Did lavender ever make for bodily
associations? Rather has it ever been that upon which
the angels of light and mercy would bear the souls
of men to a place of mercy and peace, in which there
might be experienced more the glory of the Father.

What Cayce was saying is that scent can alter our per-
ceptions and take us to other realms or dimensions. If we
look closely at the Bible and other historical writings, we
see that this message has been trying to come through for
some time. Australian scientist Dr. Michael Stoddard cur-
rently researches the effect of scent on the human mind.
He believes that ancient man understood that scent could
awaken sexual energy, opening the door to ecstatic energies being released. He also believes that the ultimate aim
was to open the doorway to higher states of consciousness. All cultures have used scent in rituals for spiritual
connection, purification, and magic. To find out more
about this aspect of scent, we have to go back to the

original researchers in this area.

THE ANCIENT TEMPLES

It is hard to find detailed information about the really ancient civilizations. But one thing is clear: Whenever new information is uncovered, you can be sure that scented material will be mentioned. Archeological evidence from the Indus Valley suggests people prepared aromatic oils more than 4,000 years ago, and that is only as far back as we can peer. But the cultures that we do know about have had quite a love affair with the pleasant-scented flowers and resins of nature.

Evidence has shown that both the Sumerians and Babylonian cultures in the Fertile Crescent burned incense. The Sumerians were fond of juniper berries, and it is believed that they used this holy smoke in their temples as an offering to the goddess Inanna, even before the Egyptians. Later, the Babylonians continued this ritual, but burned incense on altars for Ishtar instead. During this period, juniper was very common, but other scents were used, too. As trading became wider, unusual scents from far-off lands came into use. Records show that late in their history, the Babylonians used more than 1,000 talents of frankincense during a single religious ceremony. A Babylonian talent was about sixty-seven pounds, which gives you an idea how much scented material was used and how much it was valued.

EGYPT AND THE SPREAD
OF TREE WORSHIP

From Egypt, papyrus manuscripts dating from the reign of Khufu, twenty-sixth century B.C., record the use of medicinal herbs, but another talks of "fine oils, choice perfumes, and the incense of temples, whereby every god is gladdened." Perfuming the body was important for the living, as well for the dead, on whom were used aromatic gums, spices, and oils such as cedar, cinnamon, and myrrh, in embalming.

In fact, the use of imported frankincense, sandalwood, myrrh, and cinnamon was one of the most important reasons for travel. The pharaohs demanded these scented treasures as a tribute from conquered peoples. Often, aromatic woods and plant perfumes were valued even more than the gold traded for them because the Egyptians believed the gods and goddesses had to be appeased with these scents. For this reason, much time and energy was spent in searching out new sources of the coveted scented materials. The ability to procure these scents also enhanced power and position in society. One powerful Egyptian queen, Hatshepsut, was reported to have launched a huge expedition to seek out new sources for myrrh and other rare spices. The success of her trip assured her place at the royal palace.

The need for large amounts of scented materials was constant. Aromatic plant materials were given as state tributes, donated to specific temples, and kept burning at altars. Each morning, statues were anointed by priests with scented oils, and every temple activity—and even the crowning of the pharaohs—had to be marked with the smoke of incense.

This smoke from scented material also was believed to carry the people to the other world, the land of the dead. The Book of the Dead, a collection of holy teachings written down by Egyptian scribes, describes some of their magical and religious rituals in which incense was used.

In one ritual-rich funeral ceremony, an incantation was recited four times, part of which stated, "The fluid of life shall not be destroyed in thee, and thou shalt not be destroyed in it. Let him that advanceth advance with his Ka (soul) . . . "

The instructions then advised the priest to pour water from a vessel in which two grains of incense had been dissolved. More incantations exhorted that the heart would not be stopped, that cleansing would happen. Then five grains of Nekheb incense were offered. More incantations told that the deceased had been cleansed and purified with this incense. Through this purification, the person was established among the gods. Later in the texts, other offerings are described. Some were aromatic unguents and oils: "O ye Oils, ye Oils, which are on the forehead of Horus, set yourselves on the forehead and make him smell sweet through you." Cedar oil and Libyan oils of finest quality are mentioned. They had to be the best, since their scents enabled the prayers and words to be heard by the gods.

In other areas of the texts, the cleansing and purification of boats with natron and incense are described.

Here's an interesting piece of the text describing the entering of the Hall of Maa:

"The Osiris the scribe of Ani, whose word is truth, saith: I have come unto thee. I have drawn nigh to behold thy beauties. My hands are extended in adoration of thy name of Maat (Truth). I have come. I have drawn nigh unto the place where the cedar tree existeth not, where the acacia tree doth not put forth shoots . . . Now have I entered into the habitation which is hidden, and I hold converse with Set (god) . . . The Tchatchau Chiefs of the Pylons were in the form of Spirits . . . When I smell his odour it is even as the odour of one of you. And I say unto him: I the Osiris Ani, whose word is truth, in peace, behold the Great Gods . . . I have been in the stream to (to purify myself). I have made offerings of incense.

If I am not mistaken, it sounds as if someone had

entered an altered state and was describing what they had seen there. Notice that the scents of nature and incense have not been left out.

The Egyptians became renowned for creating incense and for using scented oils. To extract the scents from the plant materials, they soaked them in fats or oils. Their most famous scent, called *kyphi*, was mentioned in the writings of many ancient philosophers. Plutarch wrote that the scent of it was a balm to the mind, easing one into sleep and bringing on good dreams.

Looking deeper into the beliefs of the Egyptians, one finds that trees were very much revered. It is interesting to note that the scents most used in ritual, do come from trees. Osiris was an important deity and considered to be, among other things, a tree spirit. When he was betrayed by his brother and killed, Isis hid his body in a hollowed pine tree, where eventually he was resurrected. A pine cone often appears on monuments as an offering to Osiris. We know now that pine and other conifer species are useful specifically for the bronchial system. The scent of pine can help breathing. The breath of life? Think about it. Why do we love to go to the mountains? Often, it's the pine-scented air! We breathe deeply and feel at peace.

Other sources site the belief that Osiris's spirit resided in sycamore and cedar trees. In tombs, Osiris's mother, Nut, is portrayed as standing within a sycamore, pouring out a drink for the benefit of the dead. In certain temples, a ritual, whose meaning can only be guessed at, has worshippers placing statues of the god upon tree branches for seven days. In inscriptions, Osiris is referred to as the "one in the tree." On some monuments, he appears as a mummy, covered with a tree or plants, with a tree springing up from his grave.

This tree worship may not be worship at all, but the portrayal of the scent obtained from the trees, which was so important in the carrying out of religious ceremony.

From this example, we see the spread of belief about the importance of trees down through the centuries. Perhaps, like the childhood game of whispering in the ear of a neighbor, who whispers in another's ear, until the story returns to the originator in a completely different guise, tree worship was passed from culture to culture until the original meaning became lost.

The European cultures embraced tree worship heartily. The Druids, especially, were quite famous for their love of oak and holly trees. And even to this day, our use of Christmas trees in connection with religious celebrations had its beginnings from these far-off times.

In ancient Germany, whose primeval forests were vast, it was natural that trees featured prominently in their stories, and many of their folktales abound with magical forests. Not surprisingly, research has found that the Teutonic words for temple and sanctuary, in reality, meant wooded grove. So the original temple was, in fact, a place where living trees grew. To show you how much trees were revered, ancient German laws imposed a horrible death on anyone who dared to peel the bark of a living tree. The culprit's navel was cut out and nailed to the naked tree, while he or she was made to walk around the tree, embracing the tree with their intestines.

The Greeks and Romans were lovers of trees, too. At the sanctuary of Aesculapius at Cos, cypress trees were cut only under penalty of 1,000 drachms. Since the trees were believed to contain spirits, ancient man believed that the trees also could speak to them.

The Ojibway tribe of North America very seldom cut living trees, for their medicine men taught them that a wailing would come from trees that were felled. The Great Spirit that resided in the trees would be hurt. Many Native American tribes used trees medicinally, such as the use of the aspen tree for colds, flu, and allergies, and the willow to ease pain. They also burned aspen wood incense in their spiritual ceremonies.

In the Moluccas Islands, when the clove trees are in blossom, they are treated like pregnant women. No one is allowed to approach the trees in such a way as to alarm or frighten them.

There has always been a strong belief that trees are powerful in some way. Magical wands were made from almond branches, and stands of Juniper were deemed sanctuary, because the trees were thought of as so protective. Cedar has always been the symbol for cleansing. The fig is a symbol of enlightenment. Sandalwood is often mentioned as the wood of divination.

OTHER SCENTS, OTHER LANDS

Although trees figure very strongly as scents to use in promoting altered states, other scented plants have been used, too. Religious ritual and physical healing often were entwined, with the priests or shamans using the plants to ask the gods for healing powers as well as other powers. In medieval Europe, peasants depended upon monks for medical care. The monks' blooming herb gardens grew lavishly, and many monks specialized in the art of healing, as well as prayer.

Many examples of Native American shamanism show that, though tribes had varying rituals, their basic beliefs were the same. In addition to their religious rituals, the shamans also used plants for healing purposes. Smudging with sweet grass and wild sage (mugwort family of artemesia) was used to fumigate participants for cleansing purposes and to invoke the help of beneficial deities. It was a belief, especially among the Omaha and Ponca tribes, that the scent of the wild sage purified by dispelling negative energies and protected those who used it from harm by negative powers. In many of the tribes, drums, rattles, and the smoking of tobacco or peyote were used so the shaman could "spirit travel" to seek out the soul of a sick person in order to rescue and heal it.

CHINA AND INDIA

China has an old and rich history from which we can glean information. The earliest record uncovered is the text called the "Yellow Emperor's Book of Internal Medicine." It lists several aromatic remedies. In one, a mixture of opium and ginger was used in the religious ceremonies. Borneo camphor is still used in China for ritual purposes.

In Tibet, medicine was the domain of the religious lamas before the Chinese invasion of 1959. The lamas used meditation and mantras to energize the herbal medicine to increase its effectiveness. Even the herb harvests were carefully timed according to astrological influences, so that the highest vibratory qualities were assured. Juniper sprigs are still burned in Tibetan temples as a form of purification.

The ancient texts of India, the Vedic literature which dates to 2000 B.C., list more than 700 aromatics as being used, including cinnamon, myrrh, and sandalwood. The Indian word for smoke, *atar*, also has a double meaning pertaining to scent: wind, odor, or essence. The Rig Veda also discusses the use of odor for spiritual as well as physical healing.

GREEKS AND ROMANS

The early civilizations of Rome and Greece sailed the high seas in search of treasures—including highly prized scents. Their daily life revolved around treasured scents. In Greece, it was believed that scent sprang from the goddesses and gods themselves, and that it pleased them when worshippers honored them with scents. Aromatic rituals included anointing the deceased, burning incense on altars, and using scent to perfume their bodies daily. The Greeks built open-plan houses so that central herb and flower gardens would scent the air when the plants bloomed. They even crowned their Olympic champions with chaplets of scented bay leaves.

Rose was most popular, and heads were often anointed with this particular scented oil. In fact, the perfuming profession was deemed a prestigious job, and some perfumers even became famous, such as the celebrated Megalus. But scent was not relegated to only perfumery. There also were mystic beliefs surrounding scent. The oracles, including the most famous one at Delphi, were the first places of Grecian temples, holy sites at which priests and priestesses were believed to be able to talk with the gods and goddesses. At Delphi, the priestess would speak in trance after sitting above a crack in the rock. From this crack in the ground, a vapor is believed to have risen from underground streams and caused trance states, but it is recorded that incenses were also burned. Apollo's prophetess was said to eat of the sacred laurel and was fumigated with it before she prophesied.

In fact, divine inspiration has always been associated with the use of plants or trees. Hindus speak with their gods by kindling a fire with twigs of sacred cedar. The Dainyal or sibyl placed a cloth over her head and inhaled a thick, pungent smoke until seized with convulsions. In Uganda, the priests get inspiration from their gods by smoking a pipe of tobacco until, worked into a frenzy, the gods begin to speak through them. In Madera, an island off Java, the spirit mediums are more often female, and they prepare for the reception of the spirit by inhaling fumes of incense, sitting with their heads over a smoking censor. In Hawaii, fragrant flowers were offered to the gods in leis, and that is how the custom of offering flowers to honored guests came about.

Scent is a very integral part of religious life and ritual. It's safe to say that its use wouldn't have been this extensive or have lasted this long unless there was a good reason behind it. The fact is, scent *can* work magic for us.

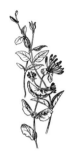

3

The Scented Veil

And the Priest, with those gathered in and about the passage
that led from the varied ascents through the pyramid, then
offered there incense to the gods that dwelt among those in
their activities in the period of developments of the peoples.
Edgar Cayce Reading 378-5

THE JOURNEY TO psychic and spiritual development is
incomplete if we don't include the information given by
America's most famous psychic, Edgar Cayce (1877-
1945). Cayce gave several readings that contained important information on the subject of scent and how it affects
the human mind and body. Today's research in aromatherapy is beginning to bear his information out, exciting
news when you realize his readings were recorded more
than sixty years ago and that science is only just now
catching up to it!

During the sixteenth and seventeenth centuries, the perfume industry underwent tremendous growth in France. But it was only in the early part of the twentieth century that essential oils began to be investigated in an empirical way for their effects on the human body and mind. It was then that the term aromatherapy was coined by Frenchman Rene-Mauice Gattefosse, a chemist, researcher, and perfumer. He was fascinated by the dermatological effects of the essential oils. In 1937, he published the first book on the subject, *Aromatérapie: Les Huiles essentielles hormones végétales,* which wasn't translated into English until much later. It really wasn't until the mid-fifties and early sixties that the United States began to see material published on the subject of aromatherapy. Even then, the information was limited, but the 1990s brought an explosion of information dealing with scent and its effects on mind, body, and spirit.

Today, fragrance trades sponsor much of the research dealing with the psychological effects of scent on animal and human brain wave patterns. They have found that when human subjects inhale aromatic vapor, even at such low levels that the scent can't be consciously detected, brain wave patterns are altered. When an essential oil known as a sedative was used, a rhythm showing calmness was produced. A stimulating aroma caused an alert response. It is believed that these responses trigger releases of certain neurochemicals (serotonin, endorphins, and noradrenalin), thus producing the various physical responses in the body and brain.

Exciting new research also is proving the effects of scent on the human body/brain. In April 2000, the first study on assessing the effects of odor on performance was done, sponsored by the Olfactory Research Fund. It revealed consistent and reliable effects on a person's positive mental condition during exercise and performance from using peppermint essential oil. Led by Dr. Bryan

Raudenbush, assistant Professor at Wheeling Jesuit University, Wheeling, West Virginia, it provided significant results that peppermint odor enhanced performance, made subjects feel more energetic and invigorated, and resulted in less frustration and fatigue after the exercise than when subjects were presented with other odors. Other studies have indicated that odor can positively affect one's mood, stress, work performance, sleep, and sexuality.

Such research has opened a door to an explosion of product development opportunities on scent in the twenty-first century. I see this as an area that will continue to expand and excite. Only a few days ago, I heard mention of a company that is preparing to digitize scent and use it through computers to enhance the computer experience. We may soon be able to smell a rose when someone e-mails a card, to sniff the scent of chocolates before we purchase them online, to use scent to wake us up and refresh us while working at the terminal, or to make virtual reality programs all the more real. While I don't understand how digitized scent will work (will they use true essential oils or synthetic versions—and will we buy "scent cartridges" like ink cartridges?) It is exciting to see all this interest in scent. It has expanded my own thinking about the future of how scents may be used.

The Edgar Cayce readings described this potential decades ago. In one of Cayce's readings on the subject of scent, he said, "For, there is no greater influence in a physical body (and this means animal or man . . .) than the effect of odors upon the olfactory nerves of the body." (274-7)

He was right on target. We know that scent is the only one of the senses that directly accesses the brain. When we inhale scent vapor or gases, they enter the body via the nose and breath. The olfactory hairs pick up the tiny scent molecules and bind them to receptors. Messages are immediately sent along neurons to the olfactory bulb, then to the limbic portion of the brain. Because the molecules of scent are so tiny, they also are readily absorbed by the skin, entering the bloodstream and again hitting the brain in record time. In one study done on caged mice, rosemary scent was introduced. Their subsequent blood samples contained a substantial proportion of one of the chemicals present in the inhaled essential oil, proving that the volatile phytochemicals *can* gain access to the bloodstream. A test you can do yourself will prove the powerful quickness of absorption. Rub a freshly cut clove of garlic on the bottom of your foot. See if the odor on your breath is not detected within 15 minutes.

It is the mysterious limbic area that the scents target. This "old brain" or "primitive brain" is where our emotions and memory, moods and sexual urges originate. I believe it is also here that the doorway to altered states lies.

Cayce also suggested that meditators could enhance their meditational states if they woke themselves at night, about 2 a.m., to practice. This, he said in a reading, is when the body is in a particular vibratory pattern " . . . where it is between the physical, the mental, and spiritual . . . " (1861-19) It comes as no surprise then, when we learn that researchers have found that nighttime is when our sense of smell is most acute. So when we meditate at night, we have a heightened sense of smell and, upon awakening in the middle of the night, we are at a crucial vibratory state. Put the two together, and you have a powerful combination!

I have often heard it said that vibration is life! Cayce agreed. Everything the sun touches is infused with energy: trees, stones, animals, and people. Plants, too, take in this energy of the sun, and in return, produce the essential oils that give off scent, another form of vibration. For vibration is nothing more than movement. Every atom is moving to the activity of a positive or negative force. Electricity is powerful vibration. (Cayce said electricity is akin to what we would call the God-Force:

Electricity or vibration is that same energy, same power, ye call God. Not that God is an electric light or an electric machine, but that vibration that is creative is of that same energy as life itself. 2828-4.

In other readings, he said:

Life in its manifestation is vibration. Electricity is vibration. But vibration that is creative is one thing. Vibration that is destructive is another. Yet they may be from the same source. 1861-16

. . . consider the effect of the color itself upon thine own body as ye attempt to apply same by either concentration, dedication or meditating upon these. For as has been given, color is but vibration. Vibration is movement. Movement is activity of a positive or negative force. 281-29.

Researchers are struggling to understand our sense of smell. Some believe in the lock-and-key theory; in other words, that certain odor molecules "fit" like a key into certain "locks" within the olfactory nerves. However, just in the last few years, new information has begun to be explored. Scientists are questioning how receptor neurons respond to light, to vibrations in the air, to odorant molecules, or to other stimuli. They are exploring the possibility that smell is a vibratory message that the brain interprets, something the Cayce readings set forth years before. There is also the possibility that scent and color are closely intertwined. In 1954 , an American researcher,

R.H. Wright, theorized that, since odor perception might be associated with molecular vibration, the frequencies must correspond to the infrared part of the spectrum. This parallels Cayce's view that all living matter vibrates and that all of the senses are connected to vibration.

In his book, *Vibrations* (A.R.E. Press, 1979), J. Everett Irion talked about how our senses pick up vibrations from outside influences which, in turn, set up their own vibrations or electrical impulses. He explored Cayce's readings on the subject extensively and detailed how all of our senses, including that of smell, operate through vibrational channels. Our brains then go on to interpret " . . . in light of that previously learned or being learned at present. . . . The force that creates an atom is the same as that which creates a vibration, and since the basic essences of all manifestation are one, an atom and a vibration are merely different shadows of the same unmanifested essence. Therefore, like the atom, a vibration can be defined as follows: A vibration is spirit moving according to the idea of presenting its purpose."

Dan McKenzie wrote in *Aromatics and the Soul : A study of smells* (1923), that he believed there are two types of odor perception.

According to the Cayce readings and many Eastern traditions, scent can and does stimulate the olfactory nerves within the body and, in turn, changes and raises the vibrations of that body. This is the key in the attunement process. Cayce mentioned lavender, cedar, sandalwood, and orris root in the readings specifically as aids to attunement. Cayce said that when our vibrations are raised, the kundalini energies are aroused so that they begin to flow through the ductless glands of the endocrine system or chakras: "The spiritual contact is through the glandular forces of creative energies . . . " (263-13) Our ability to enter into altered states hinges upon the raising of our vibrations. He also added that scent is merely one tool to help us accomplish this; there are many other tools. In my studies, however, I have found scent to be a powerful force when used correctly and even more powerful when combined with the other tools of enlightenment that Cayce and other mystics have used and mentioned through the ages.

These ideas are supported by a very strange fact with which professional perfumers have had to deal. An aroma or perfume may have a set recipe of particular oils to be used and the amounts to mix together, but no matter how closely the formula is followed the fragrance changes according to who mixes it—and on each person wearing the scent it will smell differently, too. Originally, it was believed that the person wearing the perfume merely changed it according to their personal chemical makeup, but there is no explanation for the changes that occur during the creation of the perfume. Recently, the idea has evolved that it is the person's vibrational energy that "blends" with the essential oil's vibrational energies, whether one wears it or mixes it. They make it their personal vibration!

In *Magical Aromatherapy,* Scott Cunningham ventured to say that plant and human energy often merge and can be used with visualization techniques to manifest certain things within one's personal life.

Pythagoras, that philosopher and brilliant mind of ancient times, believed that vibrations connect all things to each other and to the Divine. It is interesting to see that now, scientifically, we are beginning to prove these theories.

In any of the esoteric texts that teach development of psychic powers, you will find ample warnings. Cayce, too, stressed the fact that care must be taken to keep yourself in the right frame of mind when developing spiritual "gifts;" that these powers be used with care and not in a selfish manner. The reasoning behind these words of caution is easy to understand: The universe is governed by simple laws that cannot be changed or circumvented. It is illustrated in the simple saying, "What you sow, you reap." If you sow seeds of hatred and harm, these come to fruit within your fields.

The important questions to ask yourself are these: Why do I want these particular psychic abilities? Is it to grow spiritually? To heal others? To take care of my family? To create? To learn? To capture joy? To share that joy with others? These are good reasons that cannot come back to haunt you. Just be sure that you do self-checks from time to time to make sure you are staying on track. Selfishness, greed, hate, or any of the negative emotions when connected with such psychic development is sure to cause unnecessary pain and discomfort. Focusing on these negative emotions can also cause a loss of psychic gifts.

EDGAR CAYCE READINGS ON SCENT

For odors *are* necessary, else would they have been given to the rose, to the violet, to the lilac, to the clover, to those things that show the beauty of a loving heavenly Father! 1402-1

The making of a specific or definite perfume or the like for the individual would be most advisable to consider . . .
Choose the individual—make something that would be expressive of the individual . . . Then this will only needs be developed and expanded to meet the needs of various individuals . . . And the remunerations for these would be not exorbitant, but so much variation from that ordinarily indicated, and still so little of that as has been seriously considered from a metaphysical or spiritual angle in this country. 1849-3

... the odors ... the body should keep about self:
... orris and lavender.   259-8

Odors—the essence of the red clover should be
that chosen."   1981-1

Peculiar—the odor of orris root is about the entity
oft, and should be kept close; as the iris, as well as a
white flower of some kind always."   1799-1

For this body—not for everybody—odors would
have much to do with the ability of the entity to
meditate. For the entity in the experiences through
the Temple of Sacrifice became greatly attuned
through the sense of smell, for the activities were
upon the olfactory nerves and muscles of the body
itself. For there protuberances were taken away.
   As to the manner of meditation, then: Begin with
that which is oriental in its nature—oriental incense.
Let the mind become, as it were, attuned to such by
the humming, producing those sounds of o-o-o-ah-
ah-umm-o-o-o; not as to become monotonous, but
"feel" the essence of the incense through the body-
forces in its motion of body. This will open the
kundalini forces of the body. Then direct same to be
a blessing to others.   2823-3

In the [life] before this we find in that land known
as in the French period, or during those of the
Louis's—the fifteenth, and during that period when
Richelieu ruled with the greater strength. The entity
one to whom Richelieu oft went as one seeking counsel from the incenses burned during that period ...
and the entity gained and lost through this experience; gaining in the *understanding* of the influences
of incense, or of odors, or of such as are cleansed by

fire, and lost in the *application* of same as respecting the influence over men. In the present, much of that as is to be met in a karmic influence is the *proper* application of these same *influences*, as may be used for the *development* of peoples, individuals, men, women, children. In these may the entity meet, overcome, understand, excel; for especially are *some* of those of the aloe, or of the myrrh, those influences innate to the entity for weal or woe . . .

(Q) What should the entity study to develop mysticism?

(A) The effect of odor, color, harmony, upon individuals. Individual study and personal application greater than books though the books of mystics may be read—but *develop* same in *personal* experience *and* application.   1714-1

Also the odors which would make for the raising of the vibrations would be lavender and orris root. For these were those of thy choice in the Temple of Sacrifice. They were also thy choice when thou didst walk with those who carried the spices to the tomb.
                                                         379-3

Violet and violet scent with orris are the odors for the entity.   1799-1

First in cleanliness, in purifying of the body . . . that ye may be purified before thyself first and then before others. The annointing with the incense, making for the raising of that ye know as thine senses or perception or consciousness of the activities to all the faults, by comparison, as arose among others.
                                                         281-25

And lavender, odors that come from sandalwood

have a peculiar influence upon the body in the present; for these bespeak of something innate within self that bespeaks of the abilities of the soul, mind and body to revivify and rejuvenate itself as to an ideal.   578-2

The odors of sandalwood or orris and violet are well; for these, when the entity meditates, create an environment for the entity.   1616-1

Hence . . . the wearing of the stone lapis linguis would be as an aid in its meditative periods . . .

Also the odor of the peach blossom, or of those natures partaking of the sandalwood as combined with same.   1058-1

(Q) What kind of incense should I use during meditation?

(A) Cedar. And hyssop.   275-39

And it is well that self, when contemplating and meditating, surround self with the environs of an oriental nature . . . with the perfumes of the East.
                                                        355-1

Also there lies the ability within the entity for the seeking out, through associations with groups or individuals who may act in the capacity of research in a particular field of archaeology. The entity may join with such a group, through the abilities for testing peculiar types of materials or associations.
                                                        274-1

How many of those that usually open an egg that's been buried for five to ten million years can, by its analysis, tell you what its composition is, or what the fowl or animal fed upon that laid it? This body can! . . .

If there were opened a sarcophagus in the form of an activity where the feet of such an animal or man or body were chemically analyzed, as related to the odors and their active influences upon the body itself, would it not be possible to indicate as to what had been the means or activities of such a body during that experience in the earth? And as to what were the principal food values? Such abilities would lend much to many of these. In opening a tomb wherein there had been the form of classifications or activities in a temple service, it would be able to tell whether there had been such sacrifices required as the destruction of animal life or of man, or whether there [were] used the odors of flowers, trees, buds or a combination.   274-7

Odors! . . . there's a kind of ivy . . . The leaf of this the body should study in its associations, for it would make an odor that would be so unusual and effective and worthwhile, as well as being that which he should use as his omen or have about him often . . .

Does the odor of an orris compound affect every individual alike? Or does the attar of roses or the essence of clover or of honeysuckle or crabapple or the like affect the same way and manner? No. To some it would bring repellent influences; to others it would bring experiences that have been builded in the inner self . . .

For, there is no greater influence in a physical body (and this means animal or man . . .) than the effect of odors upon the olfactory nerves of the body. They have made much of developments for the body. Look at the difference in your New Englander that smells of earth and certain characters, the ring-ing of the nose, and those in other climes where they have smelt hot peppers and swamps. Watch the difference in the characterizations of the individuals, or the temperament of the same. Nothing has had much more influence than such in the *material* life.

. . . from certain characterizations of soil and climatic conditions, as well as other influences—not an ivy, and it is an ivy; its bloom is purple, its leaf is shaped round instead of oblong—as the strawberry, but it's not poisonous—and it should be sought by the body.

While the fleur-de-lis may have been as a pathological symbol, the scientific would be more from the blossom and leaf of this particular flower—as an interest for this body.   247-7

Study *all* of those of the ivy family, including what has been called the geranium. For this is of *that* family . . .

In much of thy seeking (as thy advanced thought is so determined, or accepted by many), the synthetic odors, synthetic reactions from varied forms of vegetation or grasses has been accepted; yet these are much like accepting shadows—for the *real* thing! . . .

Follow the stock from which there has been the propagation of those various plants, with all their *varied* odors.

From what did the plant *obtain* its ability to produce in the one that of lemon, in another orange, in another lavender, in another violet?

Its parent stock was given, not by man but by the very Creative Forces, the *ability* to take and make that which becomes as an essence that *responds* to or sets in vibration the olfactory influences in the mucous membranes of the body of man; determining it to be *setting* in motion that which has such an influence!

For as has been indicated, and as may be or should be worked upon or classified by man, there is the ability to make odors that will respond, and do respond, to certain individuals or groups; and many hundreds *are* responding to odors that *produce* the *effect* within their systems for activities that the psychoanalyst and the psychologist have long since discarded—much as they have the manner in which the Creative Forces or God *may* manifest in an individual!

What meaneth they of old when saying: "This hath ascended to the throne of grace as a sweet savor, a sweet incense before the Maker, the Creator," but that that within the individual is made aware of that estate which he had before he entered into flesh and became contaminated by the forms of matter in such a manner? For odor is gas, and not of the denser matter that makes for such activity in individuals' lives as to make for the degrading things.

Again, what meaneth He when He gave, "I am loath to thy sacrifices and to thy incense, for thou hast contaminated same with the blood of thy sons and daughters in the manner which thou hast led them astray."

The mixing of those things, then, became as stumbling blocks. What did Jeroboam, that he made the children of Israel to sin, but to offer rather the sandalwoods of the nations or the Egyptians that made for the arousing of the passions in man for the gratifications of the seeking for the activities that would satisfy his own indulgence, rather than the offering of those things that would make for the *glory* of the Lord's entrance into the activities of the individual?

What bringeth the varied odors into the experience of man? Did lavender ever make for bodily associations? Rather has it ever been that upon which the angels of light and mercy would bear the souls of men to a place of mercy and peace, in which there might be experienced more the glory of the Father.

Yet what bringeth mace and allspice and the various peppers but that which would arouse within man that of vengeance? Why?

These are of those influences that build such in the experience . . .

Hast thou ever known the odor from a flesh body of a babe to be the same as the odor from a body that has been steeped in the sins of the world, and has become as dross that is fit only to be cast upon the dunghill to become again that through which there may be gained those activities in a sphere of opportunity for a soul expression?

Then, just as these may answer for the varied stages of an individual development, there should be those things that make for such an activity.

Look about thee; and thou may understand how that one of the canine or cat family may—through the very spoor of its master or one of its kind—determine not only the days of its passage but the state of its being, interpreted as to its ability for procreation within its own self. This ye see and have taken little thought of.

How much more, then, may there be brought into the experience of individuals that which may answer in their preparations (body and mind), through the varied effects that may be obtained in the entity or individual entering into an activity that becometh it as a son of a living God?

Does thou put upon the body of the harlot the same that thou findest upon the altar of thy Lord?

Dost thou find upon those entering at birth the same as upon those passing at death? Far apart be these, yet it is as in every law—*just* the reverse side of the same thing!

(Q) could you give some information on the relation of the sense of smell to the other senses?

(A) These apply as has been indicated in that just given. Study these, not only from the manner in which they affect the body in the various stages of its development but from that they have reflected and do reflect in the activity of that kingdom just below thee—yet so often with the appearance of being far above many of those that have made themselves beneath the animal kingdom!   274-10

To some it is necessary . . . that certain or definite odors produce those conditions (or are conducive to producing of conditions) that allay or stimulate the activity of portions of the system, that the more carnal or more material sources are laid aside, or the whole of the body is *purified*, so that the purity of thought as it rises has less to work against in its dissemination of that it brings to the whole of the system, in its rising through the whole of these centers, stations or places along the body.   281-13

How develop the psychic forces? So live in body, in mind, that self may be a channel through which the Creative Forces *may* run . . . He, or she , that may lose self, then, for others, may *develop* those faculties that will give the greater expression of psychic forces in their experience. 5752-2

And the whole of creation, then, is bound in the consciousness of self. That influence, that force is the psychic self.

As to how same, then, may be developed within self:

Each entity enters materiality for a purpose. That all the experiences in the earth are as one is indicated by the desires, the longings as arise within the experience of that which makes for the growing, the knowing within self—*mind!* Thus does the entity, as a whole, become aware that it, itself, in body, mind and soul, is the result—each day—of the application of laws pertaining to creation, this evolution, this soul-awareness within, consciously manifested.

What is the purpose of entering consciousness? That each phase of body, mind and soul may be to the glory of that Creative Force in which it moves and has its being.

And when this influence, this growing self becomes such, or so self-centered as to lose sight of that desire, purpose, aim to be *to* the glory of its source, and seeks rather *for* self, then it errs in its application of the influences within its abilities for the application of mind within its own experience . . .

Then, as has been said: There is before thee this day life and death, good and evil. These are the ever present warring influences within materiality.

What then, ye ask, is this entity to do about, to do with, this ability of its own spiritual or psychic development; that may be made creative or may bring creative or destructive forces within the experiences of others? . . .

Desire may be godly or ungodly, dependent upon the purpose, the aim, the emotions aroused.

Does it bring, then, self-abstinence? or does it bring self-desire?

Does it bring love? Does it bring long-suffering? Is it gentle? Is it kind?

Then, these be the judgements upon which the entity uses those influences upon the lives of others.

Does it relieve suffering, as the abilities of the entity grow? Does it relieve the mental anguish, the mental disturbances which arise? Does it bring also healing—of body, of mind, to the individual? Is it healed for constructive force, or for that as will bring pain, sorrow, hate and fear into the experience of others? . . .

And as these are applied, so may the entity come to apply its psychic abilities, its love, its desire, its hopes, *spiritualized* in self-effacement by placing God's *glory*, God's *love*, in the place of self; bringing hope, *hope* and *faith* in the minds and hearts, the lives of others? . . .

These are the purposes, these are the desires, these are the manners in which the mental may be applied for the soul and spiritual development; and in the manner, "As ye do it to the least of these, thy brethren, ye do it unto me," saith the Lord . . . 1947-3

Part 2

Psychic Development

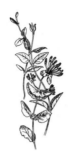

4

The Psychic Dreamer

. . . all visions and dreams are given for the benefit of the
individual, [if they would] but interpret them correctly . . .

Edgar Cayce reading 294-15

EVERY NIGHT, WE connect to our higher selves and communicate in an unlimited realm whether we are aware of
it or not. Our dreams are important doorways into our
psychic selves as many mystics, including Cayce, have
stressed. Dreams are our easiest path into another dimension, and it's easy to work with them. After all, we all
sleep every night, and we all dream every night. If you
aren't aware you are dreaming, you merely have to push
a little harder to train yourself into awareness. Dreams
are exciting theaters of the mind and are very powerful
tools if we use them correctly.

The sixth chakra handles sight and seeing. It is located in the center of the forehead and often is called the "third eye." This is the chakra with which we will be working in this chapter. Concentration on the sixth chakra when you go to bed will increase your responses.

PSYCHIC DREAMS

With very little effort, you can train yourself to remember your dreams. First, clear out the clutter in your bedroom, and make it as comfortable as possible. Purchase new sheets and bedding if you wish. Close the blinds, and try to get rid of as much distracting noise as possible. If you have to awaken at a certain time, make sure that you are awakened gently with soft music. If an alarm jolts you out of bed in the morning, you are almost sure to lose whatever memories you have from the night's dream session. Also, purchase a dream journal. It can be as elaborate as a leather-bound journal or as simple as a spiral notebook. Use a pen with a light so that, if you awaken in the middle of the night, you can record your dreams without waking anyone or having to switch on a harsh light. Another trick that works very well is to record your dreams into a tape recorder to be transcribed later into a journal. Do whatever seems to work best for you. The important thing is to record your dreams every morning. Details may not be important, but you want to get down the symbols, events, or things in your dreams that stand out to you.

The story of your dreams probably will appear to you first as symbols. As you record your dreams, themes will emerge, and you soon will be able to understand the messages that come through.

Often, dreams will tell you what to work on to improve your spiritual life, or you will be given messages about health and healing. Eventually, you will also begin to have psychic dreams, in which you will get glimpses of future events—known as precognition. This is helpful if you wish to know how to make choices in your life, if you want to know the answer to important questions, if you want to help others. You may even have retrocognitive dreams that reveal important information from the past.

You will also want to use scents that will help you to access your hidden psychic abilities and aid in psychic dreams.

SCENTS FOR PSYCHIC DREAMING

To promote psychic dreaming, you should record your dreams upon waking. To prepare yourself beforehand, obtain either a plug-in electric scent diffuser, or ideally, an electric diffuser with a built-in timer. In this way, you can have your scent diffused every two hours throughout the night. Choose which essential oil to use from the table in each section of this book or make a blend of some or all the scents. Inhale deeply about eight to ten times. Write the question you want answered on a piece of paper, and place it under your pillow, or silently ask your question three times just before going to sleep. During the night, the question and the scent will work on your subconscious mind, and you are sure to have very interesting dreams. If your dream doesn't seem to give you any answers or seems unclear, then the next night ask for a dream of clarification. Repeat the scent inhalations and always, always, always *record your dreams!*

Within a month or so of beginning to record your dreams regularly, you should begin to have important psychic dreams. Soon, you will find you can ask a question before sleep and receive an answer that night. This technique has been used for thousands of years and works well. Cayce recounted in the readings how the

ancients used temples for dream direction. A person seeking answers would go to the temple to spend one to three
nights, asking to receive answers in the form of dream
visions. In one reading, Cayce asked for an interpretation
of a dream he had had. The answer gives insight into
how dreams can be used:

The dreams or vision or both, as they are presented, represent either some development or warn-
ing, that there may be the better understanding of
the various conditions and the activities that are
active with the efforts of the body, in the attempt to
bring to others that concept which will make for
developments of individuals along the varied lines
of expressions of the individuals, or the body itself.
Ready for dreams.
(Q) [Here, Gertrude Cayce read her husband's
question to him in his trance state.] Saw myself fix-
ing to give a reading, and the process through which
a reading was gotten. Someone described it to me.
There was a center or spot from which, on going into
the state, I would radiate upward. It began as a
spiral, except there were rings all around—com-
mencing very small, and as they went on up they
got bigger and bigger. The spaces in between the
rings were the various places of development which
individuals had attained, from which I would attempt to gain information. That was why a very low
developed body might be so low that no one even
giving information would be able to give anything
that would be worth while. There were certain portions of the country that produced their own radiation; for instance, it would be very much easier to
give a reading for an individual who was in the
radiation that had to do with health, or healing; not
necessarily in a hospital, but in a healing radiation—

than it would be for an individual who was in a purely commercial radiation. I might be able to give a much better reading (as the illustration was made) for a person in Rochester, N.Y., than one in Chicago, Ill., because the vibrations of Rochester were very much higher than the vibrations in Chicago. The closer the individual was to one of the rings, the easier it would be to get the information. An individual would, from any point in between, by their own desire go toward the ring. If just curious, they would naturally draw down towards the center away from the ring, or in the spaces between the rings.:

(A) This vision is recognizable as an experience of the soul, or the *entity*, in activity. There have been various formulas or descriptions of how information for a body was obtained through these channels. There has been promised, through these channels, that there was to be a greater awakening to this entity in its field of endeavor. So in this way there is, as indicated, a way of the information being better correlated, better understood by individuals—who are through that as may be termed the attunements of the various directions, in the various portions of the country or world—of their relationship to the actual fact of seeking through the channels. As indicated, the entity is—in the affairs of the world—a tiny speck, as it were, a mere grain of sand; yet when raised in the atmosphere or realm of the spiritual forces it becomes all inclusive, as is seen by the size of the funnel—which reaches not downward, nor outward, nor over, but direct to that which is felt by the experience of man as into the heavens itself. As indicated in the rings, or the nets as of nerves, each portion of the sphere, or the earth, or the heavens, is in that place which has been set by an All Wise Creative Energy. Each may attain to those relationships by that which is attempted in the activities of an individual, a group, a class, a mass, a nation. In that manner do they create their position in the affairs of the universe. Each speck, as an atom of human experience, is connected one with another as the continuity of the cone seen, and in the manner that the nerves of an animating or living object bears upon that in its specific center, but reaches to the utmost portions of the universality of force or activity in the whole universe, and has its radial effect upon one another.

As the entity, then, raises itself through those activities of subjugating or making as null those physical activities of the body, using only—as it were (in the cone)—the trumpet of the universe, in reaching out for that being sought, each entity—or each dot, then—in its respective sphere—acts as the note or the lute in action, that *voices* that which may come forth from such seeking.

Then we find, in the classification, in the activity of those that correlate such information, those in the various spheres will naturally classify themselves— even as given in the illustration, that there will more often be the sound of help to those in Rochester than to those in Chicago. That only as an illustration. Not that there my not be as much healing to those from the one as the other, but the effect upon the individual in the environ makes for the tone which resounds from that received. See? 294-131

In this reading, Cayce discovered that his dreams were telling him how he was able to give readings of a psychic nature. There is no limit to the information you can acquire when you begin to work with your dreams.

SCENTS THAT PROMOTE PSYCHIC DREAMS

Angelica
(Angelica archangelica)

According to tenth-century tales in France, the Archangel Raphael revealed the virtues of this aromatic plant to a monk in a dream. It stimulates the nervous system, is soporific, and helps to make one more aware. It has a musky, peppery, or spicy scent.

Lavender
(Lavendula angustifolia)

It has a classic, fresh, clean scent. Helps lull one off to dreamland. It was one of the herbs dedicated to Hecate, goddess of witches and sorcerers, because of its ability to help balance the spirit with the physical. It comforts, relaxes, sedates, and purifies.

Chamomile
(Anthemis nobilis)

This apple-scented herb was held sacred by the ancient Egyptians, who dedicated it to the sun god, Ra. Later, it was dedicated to St. Anne, the mother of the Virgin Mary. It is good for balancing and calming. It stimulates the immune system while relaxing and sedating. It can be hypnotic in large doses and is inducive to meditation and sleep states.

Lemongrass
(Cymbopogen citratus)

It has been known as the scent for psychic awareness. It has an intense lemon scent. It also helps you to see the pictures in your mind when you are practicing visualizations.

REAL-LIFE EXAMPLES OF HELP
FROM PSYCHIC DREAMS

1. A divorced woman worrying over finances and how she would take care of her family dreamed of the person to contact to be hired for a job perfect for her talents and abilities.

2. A lonely woman wondered if she would ever meet "Mr. Right." After following the instructions outlined here, she not only dreamed of her future husband, but also of the hardships and happiness ahead, so that she could prepare herself for her new life. Strangely enough, the dreams seemed to "draw" him to her, and they were introduced on a blind date arranged by mutual friends.

3. A man dreamed of a mole on his arm that wouldn't stop growing. Upon waking, he went to the doctor, who diagnosed and removed a precancerous mole.

4. A young man dreamed of his mother boarding a plane that then crashed. He knew she had been planning a special trip for the last year, but when he woke, he convinced her to cancel her plans. The plane took off without her and crashed, with no survivors.

LUCID DREAMS

Sigmund Freud once mentioned what have come to be called lucid dreams:

> . . . there are some people who are quite clearly aware during the night that they are asleep and dreaming and who thus seem to possess the faculty of consciously directing their dreams. If, for instance, a dreamer of this kind is dissatisfied with the turn taken by a dream, he can break it off without waking up and start again in another direction just as a popular dramatist may under pressure give his play a happier ending.

Have you ever had a dream where you were suddenly aware that you were dreaming? Have you ever had "false" awakenings, where you dreamed you awoke, only to realize you were still dreaming? This may even have happened several times in succession. Have you ever felt paralyzed and unable to move upon waking? These are all signs that you have had or have been on the verge of having a lucid dream—a dream in which you become aware that you are dreaming while still in the dream state.

Surveys estimate that about fifty percent of people have had at least one lucid dream in their lives, so it is a very common phenomenon. Neither gender, age, nor education seem to be factors in who has lucid dreams, and they seem to be possible for all. With just a little practice, you, too, can have them. I have found them to be immensely enjoyable as well as spiritually enhancing. In some of my lucid dreams, I have been able to talk with my spirit guides, to create magical cities, to explore other worlds, to talk with deceased friends and relatives, and to face my fears. I've been able to dream myself achieving things before I actually do, to consciously practice things in my dreams so that I am more sure of my abilities in the physical!

For more than fifty years, most psychologists denied the ability of people to be able to keep their conscious awareness as they slept. These could not be real dreams, they said, but merely brief moments in the half-awake/half-asleep stage. It was only the discovery of rapid eye movement (REM) during deep sleep stages that allowed experimentation that proved the reality of lucid dreams. Keith Hearne of the University of Hull and lucid dreamer Alan Worsley performed an experiment in which Worsley used a set of prearranged eye signals to tell Hearne when he felt himself to be in the lucid dream state, thus establishing that lucid dreams not only occur during sleep but during the deepest sleep states—during REM.

There also are strong connections between lucid dreaming and out-of-body experiences (OBEs) or astral-travel states. Lucid dreaming apparently can lead to out-of-body travel.

For thousands of years, Tibetan Buddhists have practiced lucid dream states as a way to spiritual enlightenment and growth. They have developed simple, yet effective, methods for inducing such states. Lama Surya Das is one of the most highly trained American-born lamas in the Tibetan Buddhist tradition. He has studied with great spiritual masters from India, Tibet, and Asia for more than thirty years, and is the founder of The Dzogchen Foundation. He also is a poet and author of many book, including *Awakening the Buddha Within* and *Awakening to the Sacred.* Here is his method:

> When you are ready to go to sleep, relax and close your eyes. Now, concentrate on the subtle inner light behind your eyelids. Meditate into that light as if it were a vast sky or moon. What you're trying to do is "brighten" your awareness as you're going to sleep, rather than darkening it. While you do this, silently repeat a firm and strong intention to awaken within the dream, such as: "May I awaken within the dream tonight for the benefit of all dreaming, dreamlike beings." Be patient with yourself. Just do it every night, or as often as you can, and see what happens.

Here are some other tips:
- Once you realize you are dreaming, it can be hard to stay in the dreamscape, so try not to become excited.
- If you become lucid in a dream and then one of the dream characters is threatening, you may become afraid and awaken. This is a safety mechanism. It prevents those not initiated into dream study from exploring further until

they are ready. If you keep working on it, eventually, you will be able to stay calm and tell the character to disappear. Then will you be able to progress in your dream work.

PLANNING LUCID DREAMS

There are many methods for planning for and inducing lucid dreams. Perhaps the most simple method, and the one mentioned most often, is the "look at your hands" technique.

To reduce the stress of trying to have lucid dreams, you may want to plan ahead for it. Think about it during the week, and plan for it on a weekend when you have time to read and think about it. Let the idea of having a lucid dream come into your thoughts often.

To use the hand technique, look at your hands at least half a dozen times throughout the day. As you do so, ask yourself: Am I dreaming? The goal is to try to be aware enough later, in the dream, to see your hands and when you do, to again ask yourself if you are dreaming. Instantly, you will know you are. Once you are lucid in the dream, try to keep that awareness. As you do this and become comfortable in this dream state, you will eventually be able to direct your dreams in any manner you want. If you begin to feel you are losing your awareness, try spinning your body in the dream. As you twirl around, you should become more firmly grounded in your dream.

Upon retiring for the evening, place your scented essential oil blend in an electric diffuser. Time it to go off about four hours before you are to awaken. Research has shown that lucid dreams most often occur late in the sleep cycle.

Then repeat to yourself as you fall asleep: I am aware and awake.

SCENTS THAT PROMOTE LUCID DREAMS

Aniseed
(Pimpinella anisum)

It's role has been to keep out nightmares, avert evil, and generally protect. The ancient Egyptians used it not only for medicine, but also as a culinary spice. This scent is good for stress and fear, and is both physically narcotic and naturally stimulating. It uplifts and helps one draw away from fear. It has a rich, liqorice-like, sweet scent.

Dill
(Anethum graveolens)

This scent is helpful for keeping hold of the conscious mind. It sharpens the mind and heightens clarity. It is also good for allowing dreams to come through.

Clary sage
(Salvia scleria)

It balances as well as relaxes and rejuvenates. It intoxicates and sends off to sleep, but at the same time, it brings inner tranquility and sends away negative energies such as fear. It has been said to feed the soul and open us up to creativity and intuition. If we lack courage or have little fears, this scent will help.

THE OUT-OF-BODY EXPERIENCE (OBE)

The out-of-body experience (OBE), also called astral projection, is, perhaps, one of the most life-altering experiences there is. When the spirit or soul and its astral form escape the physical body, to explore other realms of existence, we see firsthand that we are eternal beings, without end, with endless possibilities at our command. In astral projection, the person's consciousness as well as the astral body separate from the physical body. When this occurs, the person has feelings of flying or floating. Such an OBE can result during lucid dreaming.

The late Robert Monroe, author and founder of the Monroe Institute, may be the most well-known out-of-body experiencer in the Western world. His many out-of-body travels and his extensive documentation of them serve as a guide for others to follow. Monroe documented accounts of OBEs in ancient Egyptian texts and from other cultures. He maintained that OBEs are natural experiences to human life, sometimes occurring during severe stress or illness, or near death. He also noted that dreamers often report "leaving the body" and that many vivid dreams of flying are actually naturally occurring instances of OBEs. Monroe taught that, with some practice, OBEs can be controlled and experienced deliberately.

Why would anyone want to control and cultivate this experience? It opens the door to great discovery, to exploring beyond the limitations of the physical body and world. Some of the benefits reported by experienced OBEers include explorations into what they believe is true reality; firsthand, verifiable evidence of our eternal natures; increases in psychic abilities; personal development; enjoyment of imaginative powers; enhancing creativity and a sense of adventure; the ability to experience and explore past and future lives; spontaneous healing; and increased spirituality.

When one practices out-of-body travel, the sense of reality can expand from mere day-to-day existence to include many dimensions, varied worlds, self-created universes, and the spiritual realms. Research has confirmed that astral travel stimulates certain areas of the brain; most importantly, the pineal gland. Interestingly, researchers have found evidence of this gland's activation at death and in near-death experiences. Many OBEers also experience enhancement of their psychic talents, perhaps because OBE opens and balances the chakras. Some of the psychic abilities that seem to be the most enhanced include the ability to see auras, telepathy, prophetic talents, and precognition. As for healing, there have been reports of out-of-body travelers concentrating on certain areas of others' bodies and causing healing to take place. Finally, nonphysical and spiritual beings often are encountered during OBEs and can be worked with to guide one on the spiritual journeys. Some even report encounters with the Universal Mind or God. For some people, just being able to travel and learn as a diversion is a reason to try it; it is the ultimate of altered states, for it is actually being set free into the great beyond.

Here too, we find that scents can help us on our trip. Several essential oils can aid one in the journey.

SCENTS THAT PROMOTE ASTRAL TRAVEL

Purchase these herbs, dried, from your local health food store or herbal catalog.

Mugwort
(Artemesia vulgaris)

In the Middle Ages, the rumor was that this was the herb that John the Baptist wore as a girdle in the wilderness. It had many magical connections. It was believed that it would prevent travelers from being fatigued and also that it repels evil spirits. It is *the* herb for helping one develop powers of astral travel. It enables psychic dreams and awareness. The essential oil is dangerous, but you can use the dried herb safely for inhalations. An easy-to-grow herb.

Hops
(Humulus lupulus)

Use the strobile (the flower from the female plant). Use fresh strobiles or recently dried. Replace every few months; the older the strobiles, the more stimulating (not very good if you are trying to sleep).

Hops contain lupulin, a bitter aromatic that is mildly sedative, inducing sleep without any side effects or headaches. Depresses the higher nerve centers. Do not use if you suffer frequent depression. Tranquilizing and helpful in loosening of the connection of the spirit with the physical.

An easy vine to grow if you want to keep your own supply so that you can be sure of the herb's freshness. Don't keep dried strobiles longer than one year.

Marjoram
(Origanum marjorana)
Use the leaf and stem. An herb that encourages sleep and peacefulness. It is sedative and helpful in easing stress from everyday life. It will help you to release your over-attachment to the physical and so let your natural astral abilities come through. Over-inhalation will put you out immediately, and you won't remember your astral flights, so don't overdo on it. It is warm and penetrating.

Deerstongue
Also called vanilla leaf
(Liatris odoratissima)
This herb, with its pleasant, vanilla-like fragrance, helps to aid in psychic awareness. It makes the senses keen.

Sweet woodruff
(Asperula odorata)
Similar results as with deerstongue—and similar sweet, vanilla-like scent. Traditionally used in dream pillows. It gives a feeling of peace and happiness. Also aids awareness.

THE DREAM FLIGHT

Becoming an astral traveler takes much work and determination. Though we may do it many nights as we sleep, the trick is to become aware of what we are doing, and in turn, become able to control what we are doing.

The scents to use to aid in becoming aware and in control of astral travel are psychically stimulating as well as highly relaxing.

To make having an OBE easier, craft a "dream pillow." These little packets of scented herbs have traditionally been used to help insomniacs fall asleep, but you will use a pillow crafted specifically with astral travel in mind. Cloth tea bags with drawstrings make perfect packets, or you may sew your own cloth bags on three sides and tie them shut after the mixture of herbs are added. When filled, the bags still need to be relatively flat to slip between the pillowcase and pillow. As you sleep, the scents will do their work. In addition to the herbs mentioned here, you also may add a few drops of chamomile and lavender, which are pleasant all-around scents for helping one sleep. Use all the scents, or merely two or three, but make sure you add mugwort, as it is especially useful to promote astral states.

Stuff a small bag (no larger than 4 inches x 4 inches) with dried herbs. Add a few drops of the essential oils mentioned, if you wish, and seal the bag. Place this bag between the pillowcase and pillow. Make sure you have a nightlight plugged in or a very low light on a table away from the bed. On going to bed the night you wish to experiment with astral travel, have a timer set so you will awaken at about 3:00 a.m. Get up, get a drink of water, go to the bathroom, stretch, and then return to bed.

Take eight to ten deep breaths. Close your eyes. Imagine, for a few moments, a swirling energy that begins at your feet and spirals upward. Have it gather at the top of your head, in your forehead, then swoosh down and begin swirling upward again. Do this for several minutes. Now imagine yourself tingling all over. Your toes tingle, your arms tingle. Keep imagining all this until you really feel the sensations. Breathe deeply. When you are tingling all over, imagine that you are flying to some destination that you know: a friend's house, a park you like, or a country or person you are attracted to. Keep imagining the story of what happens and where you go as you drift off to sleep. In your mind, keep repeating: *I am aware, and I will remember.*

It may take several sessions, but eventually, you will have an astral "dream" which isn't really a dream at all. You will actually be traveling astrally. Be sure to record your dreams upon awakening!

Another method of promoting OBEs through scent is by anointing the forehead with oil.

To make the oil, mix:

> 2 drops clary sage
> 2 drops lavender
> 1 drop nutmeg
> 1 drop yarrow
> 1 drop benzoin tincture

Add these drops to ¼ cup of olive oil. Shake. Make the mixture and place in a closed container so it will be ready for use.

Use this upon retiring to bed. Rub over the bridge of the nose, in the area of the third eye (middle of the forehead).

REAL-LIFE EXAMPLES OF ASTRAL TRAVEL

1. A young woman traveled the dimensions to visit her past lives. She got to ask questions and learned a great deal about the lessons she needed to learn. In one of her lives, she visited an ancient life in Greece as a soldier.

2. In one of his first OBEs, a man dreamed of climbing a monastery to a tower, where he stood at the edge and noticed the startling colors of the leaves on the trees. Suddenly, he spread his arms and swooped off the ledge. He flew out across the valley and realized he actually was in astral flight. The scene changed to a familiar valley, and he realized he had traveled to his old farm in another state. He could tell his house had been painted a different color and was able to verify this fact after waking.

3. After many startling dreams of flying, a woman noticed that she had a silver cord attached to her. When she awoke, she read more about astral travel and learned that one of the signs of astral travel is that one is linked to the physical body with a silver cord.

SPECIAL NOTES ABOUT ASTRAL TRAVEL

1. If you find yourself jolted awake, like a shock, this is a sign that you have been suddenly drawn back to the physical body.

2. Remember that you will be attached to your physical body by a fine silver cord. This cord is broken (contrary to rumor) only at the death of the physical body. The astral body cannot break the bond by flying "too far" or going through walls and that sort of thing.

3. Your astral body *can* pass through solid material, although this may not occur during your first few projections. With experience, you will gain confidence to travel far and wide. In your first OBE, you wish only to float up to the ceiling and look down on your sleeping body (always a shock the first time). Remember that, in the astral, thinking makes it so. So if you want to go somewhere or visit someone, just think of it or them, and you'll go. Whenever you think of your body, you will be drawn back to it and, possibly, back inside it, thus ending your

session, so it's best to keep your mind on the task at hand.

4. Don't be surprised to see other people going about their business but unable to see you. And don't be afraid if you see other astral travelers. You may even be able to communicate telepathically with them.

5. An interesting experiment is to have a friend select an object to place on a table near their bed. Then, for the next week or so, try to travel astrally to that friend's house and "see" what the object is. This will confirm for you that, "Yes, I'm actually out of my body!"

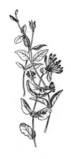

5

The Psychic Meditator

And another angel came and stood at the altar, having a
golden censer: and there was given unto him much incense,
that he should offer it with the prayers of all saints upon the
golden altar which was before the throne.

And the smoke of the incense, which came with the
prayers of the saints, ascended up before God out of the
Angel's hand.   Revelation 8:3-4

THE MOST EXCITING results can be obtained when one
practices meditation, particularly the ancient, revered
form now called the kundalini meditation.

Many secret societies and mystical texts talk of this
form of meditation. It has been a part of many cultures
throughout history, in one way or another. Ancient texts
tell us of the body's energy system and the energy centers
that make it up, and each culture had a name for those

centers. In India, the rishis and forest yogis called them *chakras,* as we do today. The Sanskrit word means "wheel." Tibetans call them *khor-lo,* which also means wheel. In Chinese Taoist traditions, they were simply called energy centers. The Sufis called them *latifas* or "subtle ones." The Hopi Indian tribes passed down teachings of the "energy systems."

Kundalini meditation is a powerful meditation designed to awaken the energy (kundalini) that lies coiled at the base of the spine in the first chakra. Awakened, the kundalini energy travels up the body to the highest center, flooding the body with energy and releasing the psychic powers within. Such meditation has been used for both spiritual enlightenment and psychic development. Edgar Cayce's readings continually stressed the important connection between such psychic development and soul growth:

> Psychic is of the soul; the abilities to reason *by* the faculties or by the mind of the soul. And when this is done, enter into the inner self, opening self through the ideals of the meditation that have been presented through these channels, and surrounding self with the consciousness of the Christ that He may guide in that as will be shown thee; either in writing (inspirationally, not hand guided) or in the intuitive forces that come from the deeper meditation, may there come much that would guide self first. Do not seek first the material things, but rather spiritual guidance, developing self to the attunement to the psychic forces of the spheres as through the experiences in the varied activities in the varied planes of experience, but ever in the light of that promise that has been given to be known among men, "If ye love me, keep my commandments, that I may come and abide with thee and bring to thy remembrance those things

that thou has need of that have been between me and thee since the foundations of the world!" 513-1.

Kundalini meditation awakens something within each one of us, a power that, when channeled properly, can be used to help and heal. Cayce also said, "*Every* entity has clairvoyant, mystic, psychic powers . . . The intuitional, which is both clairvoyant *and* psychic, is the higher development; and this may be applied in the teaching . . . " (1500-4)

What kinds of psychic powers can be awakened? Mediumship or contact with the spirit world, healing, telepathy (knowing another's thoughts), psychometry (being able to read vibrations from objects), clairvoyance (seeing an event at a distance as it happens), clairaudience (hearing messages), and automatic writing. Other powers and "gifts" are detailed in yogic writings, including enlightenment (a superconscious state of mind or being at one with God) which brings true peace and happiness. It is said that the powers of all the senses are heightened, and that one can know future and past incarnations, visit other worlds and solar systems, be able to levitate, and be able to vanish from sight at will.

USING SCENTS IN MEDITATION

In meditation, you can use diffusers and incense to increase your abilities to enter into the altered state that enhances the release of the kundalini energy.

Incense comes in many forms; there are cones, sticks, and powders. All have one purpose: to burn and send scented smoke into the air. It has been a popular form of aromatic scenting for thousands of years and used in many religious rituals. Incense is easy to use and works well in enhancing meditation. In ancient Egypt, incense balls were made of resinous and fragrant material and were called *kyphi*. Here's a recipe that I have adapted from the original Egyptian recipe. I call it:

The Gate to Inner Tranquility
½ cup raisins
¼ cup powdered nutmeg
½ cup powdered cinnamon
¼ tsp. sandalwood essential oil
½ tsp. frankincense essential oil
¼ tsp. lavender essential oil
½ cup or enough red wine to moisten the mix to a thick-dough consistency. Weigh this and add ten percent of the total dough weight in saltpeter or potassium nitrate (to ignite). Mix well.

Make one-inch balls; roll these in benzoin tincture. Dry for at least three weeks, until firm. Aging improves the quality of the scent.

A special note: Make sure that when you burn your incense, it is in a heat-tempered censer, suitable for your purpose. The smoldering incense will create high temperatures and can damage furniture if not contained in a proper burner. If you have a rock mortar, that will work. You can even use a bowl half filled with sand or salt. When you light your stick or ball incense, hold the flame to the incense until you see that the tip is glowing or burning well. It should smolder and give off a scented smoke. Also, keep incense out of the reach of children or pets.

If you prefer not to make your own incense, you can purchase unscented incense sticks and add a few drops of your own mixture of essential oils. You also can sprinkle essential oils on lighted charcoal (be careful; essential oils will flame). Powdered incense can also be sprinkled on burning charcoal.

For those of you who prefer not to use the smoke

method, you can use a diffuser. The small, electric pot-pourri simmer pots will work as well as the more expensive electric diffusers that propel fine mists into the air.

Here's a recipe for a potpourri pot. I call it:

The Temple Within
4 drops of frankincense
2 drops of lavender
2 drops of Hyssop
Mix together and add to ¼ cup water in potpourri pot.

Still another method is to mix the essential oils of your choice and paint this on a cold lightbulb with an artist's brush. Let this dry, then turn the light on. As the bulb heats up, it will scent the room you are in. Last, you can add essential oils to the lamp oil or fuel. It will burn and release the scent into the air. Experiment with the amount of essential oils to add so that the scent is not too overwhelming.

Another method is to use the forehead anointing oil on page 70. Use this upon retiring to bed. Make the mixture and place in a closed container so it will be ready for use.

Cautions: Large doses of essential oils can cause headaches or nausea. It is recommended that you not take alcohol with these scents. Also, avoid their use if you are pregnant or nursing. Nor should these oils be used by children. Always exercise care in using essential oils and take them only as recommended.

ESSENTIAL OILS FOR MEDITATION

Choose one scent or a combination for a mixture to create your incense or to mix in your diffuser. Choose the scents according to your feelings about the essential oil and its effects, and also according to whether you like the scent or not. Some scents may not agree with you from past karmic associations. Don't force these scents on yourself—choose another or another combination.

Canadian balsam
(Abies balsama)
This oleoresin was used extensively by Native Americans for ritual purposes. Twigs of Canadian balsam were mixed with cedar and juniper as purification incense. All pines are good for deep breathing.

Costus
(Saussurea costus)
This has been used in India and China as incense. It's woody, musty scent is tenacious. It stimulates and grounds.

Elemi
(Canarium luzonicum)
Used throughout the Arab and Turkish world in ancient times, its name in Arabic means "above and below." This is a shortened version of the old Kabbalistic and alchemical concept, "as above, so below," and refers to the correspondence between the spiritual and earthly realms. It encourages deep peace, combined with full lucidity. It has a light, fresh, balsamic/spicy and lemonlike odor.

Eucalyptus
(Eucalyptus globulus)
It has a harsh, camphoraceous odor with a woody undertone. It balances, clears, and stimulates. The Aborigines of Australia burned the leaves, in a form of fumigation, by seating the sick in the smoke from the fire. The powerful odor revitalizes and stimulates the whole nervous system.

Galbanum
(Ferula galbaniflua)
Used in Egypt as incense and for embalming, it is a fragrant, greenish gum resin. It was an ingredient in the famous Mendesian perfume called The Egyptian. The Hebrews used it as anointing oil. It is warming, healing, and sedative.

Myrrh
(Commiphora myrrha)
This powerful scent heals, purifies, and soothes while uplifting the spirit. It has a hot, bitter, and yet musty scent. The Vedas and the Koran mentioned its use in religious ceremony. It was one of the gifts from the Magi to baby Jesus. The Egyptians burned it every day as part of their Sun-worship ritual. It has a calming effect on the mind, instilling peace and tranquility. Moses took it with him from Egypt so the Jews could continue their use of it in their worship, so important was it to their rituals. They mixed myrrh with wine to raise their state of consciousness before religious ceremonies. It helps to release past emotional blockages.

Nutmeg
(Myristica fragrans)
Large quantities of this are hallucinogenic and excitant

to the motor cortex, so use with care. It was cultivated in Indonesia and Sri Lanka and mentioned in the fifth century. It was considered valuable and used in ungents, elixirs, and balms. According to the Doctrine of Signatures (another version of "as above, so below"), it was used as a remedy for all mental ailments, due to the seed's resemblance to the human brain. Its potential poisonous and hallucinogenic effects were first recorded in Europe in 1579 by Lobellus. It is said that the scent of the Nutmeg Islands is so powerful that the birds of paradise that inhabit the isles become intoxicated. In southern India, nutmeg is mixed with betal and snuff and taken as a euphoric. Its effects include clairvoyance and divination. The scent warms, comforts, and elevates the mind.

Rosemary
(Rosmarinus officinalis)
Sprigs were burned at shrines in ancient Greece. It was used as a fumigant in the Middle Ages to drive away evil spirits. The Egyptians used it as a ritual cleansing incense. Traces of this were found in the First Dynasty tombs. An old French name for it was "incensier," and it was burned in French churches and cathedrals. It uplifts the mind, while also dispelling confusion and giving clarity. It was a remedy for fainting. In the ancient world, it was regarded as a sacred plant, imparting peace to the living and the dead. In Asia, it was grown on tombs so an ancestor's help and guidance could communicate themselves to the living.

Sandalwood
(Santalum album)
It is one of the oldest known perfume materials, with

4,000 years of uninterrupted use. It was used in em-balming and perfumery all over the East and was a popular wood for building temples. In India, it was often combined with rose in the famous scent, attar, and used to purify body and soul and wash away sins. In Tantric philosophy, it was recommended for men only, to be used to awaken the kundalini energy and transform one to an enlightened state of mind. It was featured in ancient Chinese texts and in Tibet. In Mos-lem countries, it was placed with other scents in cen-sers at the feet of the dead, so that the soul could be carried heavenward.

Vetiver
(Vetivoria zizanoides)

It is a grass grown in India. It calms, grounds, protects, and uplifts. It is a sedative to the nervous system, while also stimulating circulation. It is deeply relaxing and known in Sri Lanka and India as the "oil of tranquil-ity." Sanskrit texts refer to it as having been used to anoint brides. It grounds; inspires a quality, deep medi-tation; and is earthy, with a smoky odor.

KUNDALINI MEDITATION METHOD

When you undertake kundalini meditation, be aware that this may require several months of practice before you obtain results. But remember that nothing of value was ever obtained easily.

Meditation is simply quieting the mind and allowing yourself to go inward. This method of meditation is spe-cific to awakening the kundalini energies, so it may be somewhat different from meditation techniques you have been taught before.

Choose a specific time that you can meditate each day. You will want to allow up to an hour for your session, so make sure it is a time when you will not be disturbed. Take the phone off the hook and tell others not to call or stop by during this hour. This meditation is best done lying down. Prepare your scent ahead of time, and have the incense or diffuser ready. You may want to use soft music or you may just want silence. You may also use an affirmation of your choice. Begin to scent the room. Wear loose clothing and lie down at your appointed time.

Your goal is to awaken the kundalini and get it flowing upward. Many yoga books have instruction on kundalini meditations, but, basically, it involves visualization and rhythmic breathing so that the chakras draw the vital force toward the top of the head.

For some, this will take some time; others may experience the effect sooner. If you need that little push to illustrate that this is all real, you can do an experiment that will immediately show you the power of the energy that flows within us. It will take the help of some friends, four or five to be exact.

Authors Walter B. and Litzka R. Gibson explained this test in their book, *The Complete Illustrated Book of the Psychic Sciences:*

> One person lies flat on his back, preferably on a couch, keeping his body rigid. Four other persons take positions, two at each side, and extend their forefingers beneath the first [person's] body at intervals from neck to ankles. All five breathe rhythmically in unison, taking in a long breath, retaining it, and exhaling at a given signal, which can come from still another person. On a designated breath—say the fifth—everyone lifts together . . . To their amazement, the four lifters bring the supine person upward on their fingertips. The effect is that the

person's body had gone weightless.

This experiment combines the kundalini force of five people and it really does work.

Because breath is so vital and important to effective meditation and activating kundalini, you must breathe correctly. As you lie there, breathe in deeply. Fill your lungs and hold your breath to the count of ten. Slowly release the breath and expel it from your lungs, from the bottom of the lungs all the way to the top—slowly, slowly. Smoothly inhale again and repeat this procedure up to five times.

Next, take a normal breath and, with your eyes closed, visualize the color red and its position among the chakras (see Figure 1, page 87): the first, or root, chakra at the base of the spine. Stay there in your mind's eye until you can see the color red. When you do so, move up to the second chakra located just above the pelvic bone, and visualize the color orange. Wait until you actually see the color orange in your mind's eye. Now move to your third chakra at the navel/solar plexus area. Visualize the color yellow. Really see the color yellow; do not try to rush it. Your heart, or fourth, chakra is next, with the color green. Remember to take your time until you really see the color green. Next comes the fifth chakra in the throat area, with the color blue. See the color blue. The sixth chakra is associated with lilac and is often referred to as the third eye located between the eyebrows. See the color violet or lilac before you move on. The last chakra is at the crown of the head, and you should visualize a golden-white light. Now, visualize your body bathed in this light, which flows down and then back again through all the chakras, making them pulsate with vibrational energy. See this for several moments.

Now begin your affirmation, one word chosen because of its special meaning to you. It can be God, or Love, or

Wisdom—whatever you choose. Silently repeat your affirmation to yourself to clear your mind of any stray thoughts. If your thoughts do stray, you can come back to the visualization. Meditate for as long as you have chosen to do so. Slowly come out, stretch, take more deep breaths, and you are done.

You will know when you have awakened the kundalini energy because there will be a powerful pulsing vibration. This energy is natural, and you are merely unblocking and repairing your chakras so that your native psychic abilities can be tapped. Practice, be vigilant, and you will obtain results. You will find that you have a great understanding that may be difficult to describe. You can ask questions in this type of meditation and get instant answers. You may even see your past and/or future incarnations, and perhaps even travel to other worlds and dimensions. In the next two chapters, you will also learn specific ways to work with the chakras to develop other psychic gifts. Study the chakra charts on pages 87-91 and they will help in your preparations.

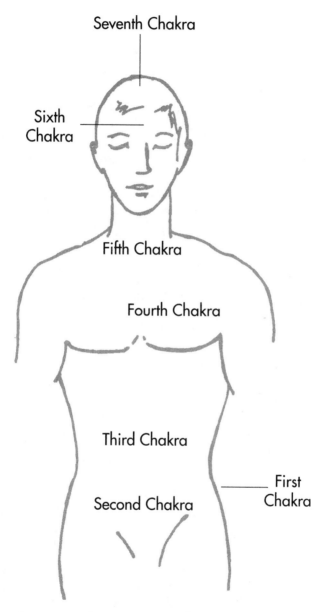

Figure 1: The Locations of the Chakras

CHAKRA CHART

First or Root Chakra
Base of spine—Red

Psychic: Your relationship to your physical body and the material world. When balanced, its energy helps to blend the physical and spiritual and eliminate what isn't needed for growth any longer. Represents earthy grounding, physical survival, sexuality in men.

Health: Governs general health and vitality. When unbalanced, you may be afraid of life, feel victimized, withdraw from physical reality, or operate selfishly. Physical symptoms include any difficulties with feet, legs, or lower back.

Second Chakra
Navel or lower area of stomach,
just above pelvic bone—Orange

Psychic: Directly related to energy flow—of blood, sexuality, and creativity. Deeply connected to the five physical senses. Female sexuality, pleasure, and desire. Governs the psychic ability of clairsentience (clear knowing).

Healing: When unblocked, you feel fully alive, spontaneous, and free of guilt. You appreciate your body. If unbalanced, you experience reproductive organ diseases, joint stiffness, and blood disorders.

Third Chakra
Solar plexus—Yellow

Psychic: Governs will, power, and raw emotions. A mastery of the physical realm and ability to master one's hopes and dreams. Relates to expression in the physical. Corresponds to emotions, psychic sight, clairvoyance, and mediumship.

Healing: When it is unblocked, you feel self-confident, have a sense of clear purpose, and pursue your dreams. Imbalances express as lack of self-confidence, insecurity about money or other physical things, and being aggressive or using power to dominate another. Digestive problems originate here.

Fourth Chakra
Thymus or heart—Green

Psychic: Relates to love and emotional well-being. Governs forgiveness, tolerance, compassion. Corresponds to psychic touch, telepathy, and loving concern. Also concerned with empathy.

Health: When it is clear, you give love unconditionally and attract others who give you an abundance of love. When it is blocked, you feel a lack of love in your life and unconnected. Heart conditions are the most common physical conditions experienced from this blockage.

Fifth Chakra
Thyroid or throat—Blue

Psychic: Associated with communication and mental creativity. Also associated with speaking in tongues, clairaudience (psychic hearing), and expression. You can hear with your inner voice, the little voice that tells you things. You will be able to read others' thoughts or instantly know the answers to difficult questions.

Healing: When balanced, you communicate easily and effectively with others in both written and verbal ways. Ability to express anger and emotions constructively. If blocked, it represents closed-mindedness and difficulties in others getting ideas across to you. Imbalances here also result in overeating, excessive drinking, and a range of respiratory diseases. There may also be problems with teeth and gums.

Sixth Chakra
Pineal or third eye—Violet

Psychic: Governs imagination, psychic perception, visualization, concentration. Also remembrance of past lives. This is the psychic center and, when unblocked, the source of intuition, psychic abilities, and ESP.

Healing: When unbalanced, you experience lack of clarity, poor eyesight, headaches and lack of concentration. If blocked, you may fear imagination, dreams, and any psychic talk. You will suffer persistent headaches, insomnia, and anxiety.

Seventh Chakra
Crown of the head—White-golden light

Psychic: Your connection to your higher self and the Divine. Higher understanding, wisdom, cosmic consciousness. Also governs the highest psychic experiences, spiritual healing, and laying on of hands. Called the "thousand-petaled lotus." Deals with astral projection and enlightenment. You will also be able to do trance mediumship.

Health: When balanced, you understand the universe and your place in it. You realize that all is one. When blocked, you feel that you are less than others, are lonely, and fear death.

THE SPIRITUAL/MATERIAL
DIVISION OF THE CHAKRAS

Spiritual:
- Seventh Chakra—Pituitary (healing center)
- Sixth Chakra—Pineal (soul memory, seat of mind)—a lesser chakra center inside the head, near the pineal. Has been deemed the soma or moon center. It is said there are many various lesser chakras in addition to the seven major ones.
- Fifth Chakra—Parathyroid/thyroid (sound, vibration, will, the Gate)

Material:
- Fourth Chakra—Thymus (heart, evolving principal, love/attachment)
- Third Chakra—Adrenals (karmic patterns)
- Second Chakra—Cells of Leydig (the door, desire, lust)
- First Chakra—Gonads (a triangle of energy where the kundalini "serpent" now rests)

CAYCE READINGS ON MEDITATION

What Meditation Is

. . . What *is* Meditation?

It is not musing, not daydreaming; but as ye find your bodies made up of the physical, mental and spiritual, it is the attuning of the mental body and the physical body to its spiritual source . . .

. . . it is the attuning of thy physical and mental attributes seeking to know the relationships to the Maker. *That* is true meditation . . .

. . . ye must learn to meditate—just as ye have learned to walk, to talk . . .

. . . there are physical contacts which the anatomist finds not, or those who would look for imaginations or the minds. Yet it is found that within the body there are channels, there are ducts, there are glands, there are activities that perform no one knows what! In a living, *moving*, thinking being. In many individuals such become dormant. Many have become atrophied. Why? Non-usage, non-activity . . .

. . . in thine own body there are the means for the approach—through the desire first to know Him; putting that desire into activity by purging the body, the mind of those things that ye know or even conceive of as being hindrances—not what someone else says! It isn't what you want someone else to give! As Moses gave of old, it isn't who will descend from heaven to bring you a message, nor who would come from over the seas, but Lo, ye find Him within thine own heart, within thine own consciousness! if ye will *meditate*, open thy heart, thy mind! Let thy body and mind be channels that *ye* may *do* the things ye ask God to do for you! Thus ye come to know Him.   281-41

Meditation, then, is prayer, but is prayer from *within* the *inner* self, and partakes not only of the physical inner man but the soul that is aroused by the spirit of man from within.   281-13

How to Meditate

(Q) Please explain . . . the steps I should take in . . . meditation . . .

(A) In whatever manner that to thine own consciousness is a cleansing of the body and of the mind . . . Whether washing of the body with water, purging same with oils, or surrounding same with music or incense. But *do that thy consciousness* directs thee! . . .

Then, meditation upon that which is thy highest ideal within thyself, raise the vibrations from thy lower self, thy lower consciousness through the centers of thy body to the temple of thy mind, thy brain, thy eye that is single in purpose; or to the glandular forces of the body as the Single Eye.

Then listen—listen.   826-11

. . . Never open self, my friend, without surrounding self with the spirit of the Christ, that ye may ever be guarded . . .   440-8

First, *cleanse* the room; cleanse the body; cleanse the surroundings in thought, in act! Approach not the inner man, or the inner self, with a grudge or an unkind thought held against *any* man! Or do so to thine own undoing sooner or later!   281-13

(Q) What is my best time for meditation?

(A) As would be for all, two to three o'clock in the morning.   462-8

(Q) [What is the best polarity for this body] as it meditates?
(A) Facing the East, to be sure.   2072-12

Then, as one formula—not the only one, to be sure—for an individual that would enter into meditation for self, for others:
Cleanse the body with pure water. Sit or lie in an easy position, without binding garments about the body. Breathe in through the right nostril three times, and exhale through the mouth. Then, either with the aid of a low music, or the incantation of that which carries self deeper—deeper—to the seeing, feeling, experiencing of that image in the creative forces of love, enter into the Holy of Holies. As self feels or experiences the raising of this, see it disseminated through the *inner* eye (not the carnal eye) to that which will bring the greater understanding in meeting every condition in the experience of the body. Then listen to the music that is made as each center of thine body responds to that new creative force that is being, and that is disseminated through its own channel; and we will find that little by little this entering in will enable self to renew all that is necessary—in Him.   281-13

For this body—not for everybody—odors would have much to do with the ability of the entity to meditate . . .
Let the mind become, as it were, attuned to such [oriental incense] by the humming, producing those sounds of o-o-o-ah-ah-umm-o-o-o; not as to become monotonous, but "feel" the essence of the incense

through the body-forces in its motion of body. This will open the kundalini forces of the body. 2823-3

[The crystal ball is] a means of concentration for those that allow themselves either to be possessed or to centralize their own spiritual activity through the raising of those activative forces in the physical body known as the centers through which concentration and meditation is accentuated by the concentrated effort on *anything* that will *crystallize* same into activity. A means for some. Rather, as has been given, let the proof come from that as may be visioned in the self. 254-7

Then, as ye begin with the incantation of the [Har-r-r-r-r-aum] Ar-ar-r-r-r—the e-e-e, the o-o-o, the m-m-m, *raise* these in thyself; and ye become close in the presence of thy Maker—as is *shown* in thyself! They that do such for selfish motives do so to their own undoing. 281-28

Benefits of Meditation

As has been given, there are *definite* conditions that arise from within the inner man when an individual enters into true or deep meditation. A physical condition happens, a physical activity takes place! Acting through what? Through that man has chosen to call the imaginative or the impulsive, and the sources of impulse are aroused by the shutting out of thought pertaining to activities or attributes of the carnal forces of man. That is true whether we are considering it from the group standpoint or the individual. Then, changes naturally take place when there is the arousing of that stimuli *within* the individual that has within it the seat of the soul's dwelling, within the individual body of the entity or man, and then this partakes of the individuality rather than the personality.

If there has been set the mark (mark meaning here the image that is raised by the individual in its imaginative and impulse force) such that it takes the form of the ideal the individual is holding as its standard to be raised to, within the individual as well as to all forces and powers that are magnified or to be magnified in the world from without, *then* the individual (or the image) bears the mark of the Lamb, or the Christ, or the Holy One, or the son, or any of the names we may have given to that which *enables* the individual to enter *through* it into the very presence of that which is the creative force from within itself—see?   281-13

(Q) Is it possible to meditate and obtain needed information?

(A) On any subject! whether you are going digging for fishing worms or playing a concerto!
                                                           1861-12

Meditation and Prayer

[Gertrude Cayce] You will have before you the psychic work of Edgar Cayce, present in this room, the information that has been and is being given from time to time, especially that regarding meditation and prayer. You will give, in a clear, concise, understandable manner just how an individual may meditate, or pray, without the effort disturbing the mental or physical body. If this can be given in a general manner, outline it for us. If it is necessary to be outlined for specific individuals, you will tell us how individuals may attain to the understanding necessary for such experiences not to be detrimental to them.

[Edgar Cayce] Yes, we have the work, the information that has been and that maybe given from time to time; especially that in reference to meditation and prayer.

First, in considering such, it would be well to analyze that difference (that is not always understood) between meditation and prayer.

As it has been defined or given in an illustrated manner by the Great Teacher, prayer is the *making* of one's conscious self more in attune with the spiritual forces that may manifest in a material world, and is *ordinarily* given as a *cooperative* experience of *many* individuals when all are asked to come in one accord and one mind; or, as was illustrated by:

Be not as the Pharisees, who love to be seen of men, who make long dissertation or prayer to be heard of men. They *immediately* have their reward in the physical-mental mind.

Be rather as he that entered the temple and not so much as lifting his eyes, smote his breast and said, "God be merciful to me a sinner!"

Which man was justified, this man or he that stood to be seen of men and thanked God he was not as other men, that he paid his tithes, that he did the services required in the temple, that he stood in awe of no one, he was not even as this heathen who in an uncouth manner, not with washed hands, not with shaven face attempted to reach the throne of grace?

Here we have drawn for us a comparison in prayer: That which may be the pouring out of the personality of the individual, or a group who enter in for the purpose of either outward show to be seen of men; or that enter in even as in the closet of one's inner self and pours out self that the inner man may be filled with the Spirit of the Father in His merciful kindness to men.

Now draw the comparisons for meditation: Meditation, then, is prayer, but is prayer from *within* the *inner* self, and partakes not only of the physical inner man but the soul that is aroused by the spirit of man from within.

Well, that we consider this from *individual* interpretation, as well as from group interpretation; or individual meditation and group meditation.

As has been given, there are *definite* conditions that arise from within the inner man when an individual enters into true or deep meditation. A physical condition happens, a physical activity takes place! Acting through what? Through that man has chosen to call the imaginative or the impulsive, and the sources of impulse are aroused by the shutting out of thought pertaining to activities or attributes of the carnal forces of man. That is true whether we are considering it from the group standpoint or the individual. Then, changes naturally take place when there is the arousing of that stimuli *within* the individual that has within it the seat of the soul's dwelling, within the individual body of the entity or man, and then this partakes of the individuality rather than the personality.

If there has been set the mark (mark meaning here the image that is raised by the individual in its imaginative and impulse force) such that it takes the form of the ideal the individual is holding as its standard to be raised to, within the individual as well as to all forces and powers that are magnified or to be magnified in the world from without, *then* the individual (or the image) bears the mark of the Lamb, or the Christ, or the Holy One, or the Son, or any of the names we may have given to that which *enables* the individual to enter *through it* into the very presence of that which is the creative force from within itself—see?

Some have so overshadowed themselves by abuses of the mental attributes of the body as to make scars, rather than the mark, so that only an imperfect image may be raised within themselves that may rise no higher than the arousing of the carnal desires within the individual body. We are speaking individually, of course; we haven't raised it to where it may be disseminated, for remember it rises from the glands known in the body as the lyden, or to the lyden [Leydig] and through the reproductive forces themselves, which are the very essence of Life itself within an individual—see? for these functionings never reach that position or place that they do not continue to secrete that which makes for virility to an individual physical body. Now we are speaking of conditions from without and from within!

The spirit and the soul is within its encasement, or its temple within the body of the individual—see? With the arousing then of this image, it rises along that which is known as the Appian Way, or the pineal center, to the base of the *brain*, that it may be disseminated to those centers that give activity to the whole of the mental and physical being. It rises then to the hidden eye in the center of the brain system, or is felt in the forefront of the head, or in the place just above the real face—or bridge of nose, see?

Do not be confused by the terms that we are necessarily using to give the exact location of the activities of these conditions within the individuals, that we may make this clarified for individuals.

When an individual then enters into deep meditation:

It has been found throughout the ages (*individuals* have found) that self-preparation (to *them*) is necessary. To some it is necessary that the body be cleansed with pure water, that certain types of breathing are taken, that there may be an even balance in the whole of the respiratory system, that the circulation becomes normal in its flow through the body, that certain or definite odors produce those conditions (or are conducive to producing of conditions) that allay or stimulate the activity of portions of the system, that the more carnal or more material sources are laid aside, or the whole of the body is *purified* so that the purity of thought as it rises has less to work against in its dissemination of that it brings to the whole of the system, in its rising through the whole of these centers, stations or places along the body. To be sure, these are conducive; as are also certain incantations, as a drone of certain sounds, as the tolling of certain tones, bells, cymbals, drums, or various kinds of skins. Though we may as higher thought individuals find some fault with those called savages, they produce or arouse or bring within themselves—just as we have known, do know, that there may be raised through the battlecry, there may be raised through the using of certain words or things, the passion or the thirst for destructive forces. Just the same may there be raised, not sedative to these but a *cleansing* of the body.

Consecrate yourselves this day that ye may on the morrow present yourselves before the Lord that He may speak through *you!*" is not amiss. So, to *all* there may be given:

Find that which is to *yourself* the more certain way to your consciousness of *purifying* body and mind, before ye attempt to enter into the meditation as to raise the image of that through which ye are seeking to know the will or the activity of the Creative Forces; for ye are *raising* in meditation actual *creation* taking place within the inner self!

When one has found that which to self cleanses the body, whether from the keeping away from certain foods or from certain associations (either man or woman), or from those thoughts and activities that would hinder that which is to be raised from *finding* its full measure of expression in the *inner* man (*inner* man, or inner individual, man or woman, meaning in this sense those radial senses from which, or centers from which all the physical organs, the mental organs, receive their stimuli for activity), we readily see how, then, *in* meditation (when one has so purified self) that *healing of every* kind and nature may be disseminated on the wings of thought, that are so much a thing—and so little considered by the tongue that speaks without taking into consideration what may be the end thereof!

Now, when one has cleansed self, in whatever manner it may be, there may be no fear that it will become so overpowering that it will cause any physical or mental disorder. It is *without* the cleansing that entering any such finds *any* type or form of disaster, or of pain, or of any dis-ease of any nature. It is when the thoughts, then, or when the cleansings of *group* meditations are conflicting that such meditations call on the higher forces raised within self for manifestations and bring those conditions that either draw one closer to another or make for that which shadows [shatters?] much in the experiences of others; hence short group meditations with a *central* thought around some individual idea, or either in words, incantations, or by following the speech of one sincere in abilities, efforts or desires to raise a cooperative activity *in* the minds, would be the better.

Then, as one formula—not the only one, to be sure—for an individual that would enter into meditation for self, for others:

Cleanse the body with pure water. Sit or lie in an easy position, without binding garments about the body. Breathe in through the right nostril three times, and exhale through the mouth. Breathe in three times through the left nostril and exhale through the right. Then, either with the aid of a low music, or the incantation of that which carries self deeper—deeper—to the seeing, feeling, experiencing of that image in the creative forces of love, enter into the Holy of Holies. As self feels or experiences the raising of this, see it disseminated through the *inner* eye (not the carnal eye) to that which will bring the greater understanding in meeting every condition in the experience of the body. Then listen to the music that is made as each center of thine own body responds to that new creative force that little by little this entering in will enable self to renew all that is necessary—in Him.

First, *cleanse* the room; cleanse the body; cleanse the surroundings, in thought, in act! Approach not the inner man, or the inner self, with a grudge or an unkind thought held against *any* man! or do so to thine own undoing sooner or later!

Prayer and meditation: Prayer is the concerted effort of the physical consciousness to become attuned to the consciousness of the Creator, either collectively or individually! *Meditation* is *emptying* self of all that hinders the creative forces from rising along the natural channels of the physical man to be disseminated through those centers and sources that create the activities of the physical, the mental, the spiritual man; properly done must make one *stronger* mentally, physically, for has it not been given?

He went in the strength of that meat received for many days? Was it not given by Him who has shown us the Way, "I have had meat that ye know not of"? As we give out, so does the *whole* of man—physically and mentally become depleted, yet in entering into the silence, entering into the silence in meditation, with a clean hand, a clean body, a clean mind, we may receive that strength and power that fits each individual, each soul, for a greater activity in this material world.

Be not afraid, it is I." Be sure it is Him we worship that we raise in our inner selves for the dissemination; for, as He gave, "Ye must eat of my *body;* ye must drink of *my* blood." Raising then in the inner self that image of the Christ, love of the God-Consciousness, is *making* the body so cleansed as to be barred against all powers that would in any manner hinder.

Be thou *clean,* in Him.   281-13

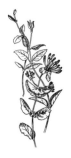

6

The Psychic Healer

Keep, in thine meditations, that of the *Christ* Consciousness being magnified *in* thee day by day . . . for we . . . so *easily* forget the promise that 'If ye abide in me, I will abide in thee,' and 'Whatever ye ask in *my* name, *believing*, ye shall have . . . ' Edgar Cayce reading 1742-4

HEALING IS ONE of the most exciting gifts with which we can be blessed in working with our psychic abilities. With it, we are able to be lights shining in the dark, pointing the way. We can be channels that aid in removing suffering and fear, for ourselves, our friends, our loved ones, and others. It is an awesome responsibility and one that must be undertaken with the greatest of seriousness.

One of the hardest things for me to learn was that we mustn't interfere with another's illness unless they ask for or agree to receive help. We don't know the circumstances behind illnesses; they can come from many aspects. Some souls choose to go through an experience of illness as a karmic lesson. Or it may be that the soul has chosen to experience an illness to help another close to them. Illness can also be caused by imbalance, negativity, or physical actions or conditions. But it can also be that the person has grown enough to be done with the experience itself and, at such times, needs a healing. Whatever the circumstance, when someone is ready to be healed, they will be prompted to seek the healing. Do not force a healing on someone who doesn't wish it. Above all, remember that you are only a channel to the healing energy that comes through you.

HEALING THROUGH PRAYER

In accepting the flow of healing power, we must become channels for it. How do we accomplish this? In the book, *Unseen Hands and Unknown Hearts: A Miracle of Healing Created Through Prayer,* by Kathy L. Callahan, Ph.D. (A.R.E. Press, 1995), the author talked about how thought can either hinder or help us. In her quest for healing for her daughter, the author explored healing prayer and, with the help of prayer groups, including the Glad Helpers at Edgar Cayce's Association for Research and Enlightenment (A.R.E.), accomplished a miraculous healing. She said:

. . . In other words, we were so caught up in the physical illusions of the disease that we could not see the reality of a miracle. While we had accepted the *idea* of a miracle as a possibility, we were giving equal credence and hence power to other possibilities as well . . . We would correctly start the miracle process, only to sabotage our own efforts by concentrating on the physical illusions of the disease and giving them equal power!

This illustrates what Cayce repeated over and over: Mind is the builder. What we have in our minds, we create. Keep this in mind when you contemplate creating a situation or healing.

There are two ways to heal through prayer. One is individual and the other is in a group.

INDIVIDUAL PRAYER

Do you want to be a channel for healing? Is it in your heart to help others who are suffering and in need? Then you have it in your heart to be an open channel of healing for yourself and others.

To perform such service, you must first meditate for your allotted period of time daily. Seek to be diligent in your meditations.

Cayce said:

No application of *any* medicinal property or any mechanical adjustment, or any other influence, is healing of itself! These applications merely help to attune, adjust, correlate the activities of the bodily functions to nature and natural sources!

All healing, then, is from life! Life is God! It is the adjusting of the forces that are manifested in the individual body . . .

The *body* is a pattern . . .

It is the cooperation, the reaction, the response made *by* the individual that is sought. Know that the soul-entity must find in the applications that response which attunes its abilities, its hopes, its desires, and its purposes to that universal consciousness.

> *That* is healing—of any nature! . . .
> *Attune* the body! 2153-6.

You attune the body through daily meditation. Choose your time to take yourself away from the world and enter into your meditations and prayer. Make it a daily thing, a special thing you do that is kept as an appointment more important than any other in your schedule.

After each meditation period, have a period of prayer—for your self and for others.

I recommend you read *Healing through Meditation and Prayer* by Meredith Ann Puryear (A.R.E. Press, 1978). This book has helped me more than any other to learn about prayer and how it works.

GROUP PRAYER

Edgar Cayce was asked during a reading whether group prayer might be more helpful or effective. He answered:

> Where two or three are gathered in my name, I am in the midst of them." These words were spoken by Life, Light, Immortality, and are based on a law. For, in union is strength. Why?
>
> Because as there is oneness of purpose, oneness of desire, it becomes motivative within the active forces or influences of a body. The multiplicity of ideas may make confusion, but added cords of strength in one become the nature as to increase the *ability* and influence in every expression of such a law. 281-24

The power of two or more people coming together to pray for healing is awesome. If one person is a beacon, two or more can become like lighthouses with a beam of healing light so powerful that one is bound to see it in a sea of trouble.

In the last eight years, I've been a part of a Search for God® study group (sponsored by the A.R.E.). We strive to meditate individually each day, and we have a healing prayer list of others for whom we pray. We also come together each week to meditate as a group and pray for others. This prayer time is the most exciting part of our study group. We have discovered that when someone is placed on the prayer list, things happen. Not everyone is healed, but a great many are. And the ones who aren't still experience positive changes.

If you decide to heal in group, here are some tips to remember:

1. Visualize together.
2. Vocalize your healing prayer.
3. Expect a miracle.
4. Thank God for His love and mercies.

HEALING THROUGH LAYING ON OF HANDS

[In meditation] When one is able to so raise within themselves such vibrations, as to pass through the whole course of the attributes of physical attunements, to the disseminating force or center, or the Eye, then the body of that individual becomes a magnet that may (if properly used) bring healing to others with the laying of hands.   281-14

The chakras play an important role in healing, as you can see from the charts beginning on page 87. If the chakras are balanced, a body becomes whole; the vibrations of healing open a way back to health. One of the reasons many people fall ill is because their chakras become misaligned; they are "unbalanced," or there are blockages that restrict the free flow of the body's energy.

Here is a method for balancing another person's chakras:

1. Visualize the healing energies flowing into your hand, up your arm, and into the whole of your body. As the healing energies flow throughout your body, ask from deep within your being that all the unbalanced vibrations within your body be completely rebalanced.

For healing to take place, you need to give yourself permission for the necessary changes to occur within your own body. You need to commit yourself—100 percent to working with the healing process. If you want to be made totally well again, you must accept total responsibility for your health.

2. After you have balanced yourself, visualize a white light of energy in your hands, building up, growing, glowing, and increasing in power.

3. Have the person who has asked for a healing to sit in a chair, with you directly behind them. Place your left hand (the negative pole) upon their forehead and your right hand (the positive pole) on the back of their head or between the shoulder blades. Ask for the healing energy to flow through you. Be open and just let time flow for a moment or two. You might have a prayer or an affirmation you like to repeat to yourself. If you are attuned, you may be led to place your hands on other areas of the body, and you will know how long to keep your hands there. You might feel a warmth or a coldness in a certain area, signaling that energy is needed there. It is interesting to note that, often, even if you don't know what the physical problem is, your hands will automatically go there during the healing. One session may be all that is needed, or more than one may be required. As you become more experienced, you will find such healing will become easier. Remember to ask Spirit for direction on how to proceed.

4. When finished, surround the person in a cloud of love and light. Bring your hands over the person's head, cupped together, and visualize healing energy flooding the person. Give thanks.

ESSENTIAL OILS FOR HEALING

Benzoin
(Styrax benzoin)

The name comes from the Arabic *lubar-jawi* or "incense from Sumatra." It has been used for medicine and fragrance for centuries. It is comforting. Fumigations of this were believed to chase away evil spirits. The essential oil warms and stimulates the heart and circulation. It imparts euphoria.

Borneol
(Dryobalanops aromatica)

It has a sassafras-like camphoraceous odor. It simulates the adrenal cortex and is tonic and antidepressant. In ancient China, it was used for embalming. In the thirteenth century, Marco Polo called it "balsam of disease." It has been used for ceremonial purposes in the East.

Cinnamon
(Cinnamomum zelanicum)

This is one of the principal spices in the mummification processes. It was mentioned in the Bible and was included in the holy ointment of Moses. In China, it is seen as a cure-all and nerve tranquilizer.

Coriander
(Coriandrum sativum)

Ancient Egyptians employed it as a remedy. The seeds

were found in the tombs of King Tutankhamaun and Ramses II. Oil from the seeds was used in religious ceremonies. It was mentioned in the Bible several times, being likened to the manna that the Lord provided the children of Israel. In India, it was used in curries and in religious ceremonies. In China, it has been used for more than 5,000 years to promote longevity. It is narcotic in excess, with a sweet, spicy, woody scent.

Cypress
(Cupressus sempervirens)

It is still considered sacred and used as a purifying incense by the Tibetans. It regulates body fluids. It has a clear, tenacious odor. There is a legend that says cypress was the wood from which Christ's cross was made. The Egyptians used it for coffin-making, and both Egyptians and Romans dedicated this tree to their gods of death and the underworld as a symbol of immortality. Its name, *sempervirens,* means lives forever, but the folk name is "tree of death." It calms, relieves stress, and is a good scent for someone going through the grieving process.

Frankincense
(Bowellia carteri)

This resin has been used since antiquity as an incense in India and China, and in the West by the Catholic Church. The scent slows and deepens breath, so it is conducive to prayer and meditation. It is a warm, rich, and sweet scent. It is restorative, heals, and is a tonic to the nervous system. When burned, it gives off a chemical called trahydrocannabinole, which is consciousness-expanding. In ancient times, its value was placed higher than that of gold. It is a spiritually uplifting scent. It has been used by many cultures to treat every ailment and burned to free the sick of evil spirits and purify the body and soul. The Jews used it as holy incense. It was burned at the Greek altars in the temples of Zeus and Demeter. In 1981, German scientists investigated the effects of inhalation and found that it did affect the mind states.

Geranium Rose
(Pelargonium graveolens)
This scent is good for melancholy. It stimulates the lymphatic system and is tonic and uplifting. It brings balance and was said to keep away evil spirits. It also has a stimulating effect on the adrenal cortex of the brain. It regulates and balances the release of hormones in the body. It stimulates the immune system and helps reduce water retention.

Juniper
(Juniperus communis)
It has a fresh, sweet odor and has been used since ancient times. It was used to anoint mummies. In Nubia, bodies were preserved with salt and juniper, and it was found in a fifth-century cemetery and Coptic monastery at Thebes. Branches of juniper were burned in Greece to combat epidemics and used as purification incense in Tibet. Native Americans burned dried sprigs in ritual cleansing ceremonies. In Britain, it was thought that smoke from juniper wood kept demons at bay. An infusion of the berries was thought to restore lost youth. It does clear away mental/emotional negativity.

Yarrow
(Achillea millefolium)

In Germany, it was known as an herb of healing. In ancient China, it was considered a sacred plant. The stems were used to make the fifty sticks for I Ching divination. In Chinese herbalism, it is thought to represent perfect balance between yin and yang energies. In the West, it is associated with divination and magic. It was said the druids used this herb to foretell the weather. It is a sweet, spicy scent that raises the spirit and aids sleep, while lowering blood pressure.

Sandalwood
(Santalum album)

One of the oldest meditation aids, sandalwood use is more than 4,000 years old and continues to this day. In India, it is combined with rose for the famous scent, attar. Just one drop massaged into swollen lymph glands under the chin will heal and balance. It has been used in Hindu purification ceremonies to wash away sin. Tantric philosophy recommends it to awaken kundalini. It helps to break ties with the past, break obsessions, build the immune system, and heal insomnia, anxiety, and psychological problems. It has a musky scent, oriental and warm.

USE OF SCENTS

During your healing sessions, you may want to burn or diffuse the scents of the essential oils listed in this chapter. It will aid in attuning the body for the healing energies to flow.

You also can magnetize the body as a healing channel and enhance the healing flow through the use of anointing oils and creams. Anointing oils have been used since ancient times. Most notably, they are mentioned in the Bible.

> The Spirit of the Lord God is upon me, because the Lord has anointed me to bring good tidings to the afflicted. (Isaiah 61:1)

> Thou anointest my head with oil, my cup runneth over. (Psalm 23:5)

> How God anointed Jesus of Nazareth with the Holy Spirit and with power . . . (Acts 10:38)

To make an anointing oil:
In two tablespoons of peanut or olive oil, add twenty-four drops of essential oil or combination of essential oils. Anoint the body by massaging the oil into the forehead at the area of the sixth chakra. You may also massage into the other chakra locations, as well as the hands and feet depending upon how you feel led.

To make an anointing cream:
Purchase an unscented cream at the pharmacy or through an aromatherapy dealer. Use twelve drops of essential oil per one tablespoon of cream. Mix thoroughly and massage as recommended above. You may even use the anointing cream on yourself in preparation for meditation.

An ancient technique for magnetizing the body in preparation for healing:
An ancient yogic technique for becoming attuned for the purposes of healing is called "magnetizing the body." It is a simple procedure that you may want to try.
Place your body in a comfortable position (or remain

in a comfortable position after your normal meditation). Relax the body completely. Think about the energy that your body contains. Visualize this energy. Feel the magnetic pulsation, first in the feet, then rising up through each part of the body. Visualize and feel the pulsation, keeping only right thoughts in your mind. You will soon feel a thrumming or humming sensation. You may also feel a fullness or electricity in the hands. Keep repeating to yourself, "My body is completely magnetized."

At the end of the session, you will feel that your body is strong, energized, and vital. You will also find your mind enlightened. Now you can practice being a channel of healing.

CAYCE READINGS ON HEALING

The *concerted* effort on the part of a group merely accentuates that as a force, or power, that may manifest in or through an individual, or as respecting a circumstance. Hence the activity must be as much on the part of one seeking aid through such a channel.   281-5

In giving counsel to those of the prayer group:

Let each seek more and more, in their daily lives, to be one of those sent by the Lord, the Christ, to someone, to awaken them to their opportunities in the love of the Christ.

Then, let each of you so act yourself that those to whom ye speak *know* ye walk and talk often with the Lord, with the Christ.

For He hath chosen each of you as a messenger to someone. Fail Him not.   281-64

As the body attunes self, as has been given, it may be a channel where there may be even *instant* healing with the laying on of hands. The more often this occurs the more *power* is there felt in the body, the [more] forcefulness in the act or word.   281-5

There are, as seen, many *various* channels through which healing may come. That as of the individual contact; that as of the faith; that as of the laying on of hands; that as will create in the mind (for it is the builder in a human being) that consciousness that makes for the closer contact with the universal, or the *creative forces,* in its experience. That which is nearest akin to that concept built. Use that thou hast, then, in hand.   281-6

When a body, separate from that one ill, then, has so attuned or raised its own vibrations sufficiently, it may—by the motion of the spoken word—awaken the activity of the emotions to such an extent as to revivify, resuscitate or to change the rotary force or influence or the atomic forces in the activity of the structural portion, or the vital forces of a body, in such a way and manner as to set it again in motion.

Thus does spiritual or psychic influence of body upon body bring healing to *any* individual; where another body may raise that necessary influence in the hormone of the circulatory forces as to take from that within itself to revivify or resuscitate diseased disordered or distressed conditions within a body.
                    281-24

There has been given by those in the orthodox manner those who *should, through* faith, laying on of hands, anointing with oil, praying over same. There is, in the broader sense, that innate in each individual that may be awakened to those abilities in their activity, are they willing to attune themselves

SEEKING INFORMATION ON

**holistic health, spirituality, dreams,
intuition or ancient civilizations?**
Call 1-800-723-1112, visit our Web site,
or mail in this postage-paid card for a FREE
catalog of books and membership information.

PBIN

Name: _____

Address: _____

City: _____

State/Province: _____

Postal/Zip Code: _____ Country: _____

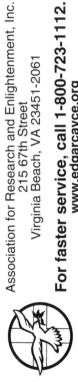

Association for Research and Enlightenment, Inc.
215 67th Street
Virginia Beach, VA 23451-2061

For faster service, call 1-800-723-1112.
www.edgarcayce.org

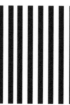

to the laws as pertain to the active forces in self's
own experience, keeping self unspotted and clean
from the world, and *keeping* that that brings according in the body that necessary for its awakening to
its own spiritual activity. Who shall do such? Such
as are called in their own experience.   262-17

. . . all illness comes from sin. This everyone must
take whether they like it or not; it comes from sin—
whether it be of body, of mind, or of soul . . . 3174-1

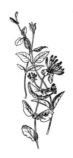

7

Enhancing the Psychic Connection

Professor H.H. Price, the Oxford philosopher and parapsychologist, suggests that once an idea has been created, it 'is no longer wholly under the control of the consciousness which gave it birth', but may operate independently on the minds of other people or on physical objects.

William G. Roll
The Poltergeist

THERE IS A riddle. It is the riddle of the ages and one that I believe we are beginning to be able to answer. If all of life contains vibratory energy—people, plants, and the Earth itself—then can we combine these energies if we know how to harness them and direct them?

The Egyptian Sphinx stands, mutely guarding the pyramids. It seems to ask another riddle: What am I guarding? In *Pyramid Power* (Warner-Destiny, 1974), authors Max Toth and Greg Nielsen put forth the theory that the pyramids are not only accumulators of energies but also resonators able to focus energies of the cosmos like "a giant lens." Experiments have shown that pyramids are able to do amazing things (energize water to create healing waters, enhance meditational states, mummify or preserve any thing placed within, and more). Apparently, the shape of the pyramid serves as a collector of outside energies, as well as an amplifier of whatever energy source is inside.

Those who have studied dowsing and ley lines know that the pyramids are a part of this pattern of energy "conduits." If we are assuming correctly, it seems the ancients recognized a pattern of lines across the earth— ley lines—which they marked with temples and other holy shrines. The Egyptian and other pyramids serve as conductors and transformers of the energy and have been linked to these lines and cosmic positionings.

Herefordshire businessman Alfred Watkins was the first to notice the pattern of ancient holy sites. In 1925, he published *The Old Straight Track* and described his first thoughts at the discovery:

> Imagine a fairy chain stretched from mountain peak to mountain peak, as far as the eye could reach, and paid out until it reached the "high places" of the earth at a number of ridges, banks and knolls. Then visualize a mound, circular earthwork or clump of trees, planted on these high points, and in low points in the valley other mounds, ringed around with water to be seen from a distance. Then great standing stones brought to mark the way at intervals and on a bank leading up to a mountain ridge or down to a ford, the track cut deep so as to form a guiding notch on the skyline as you come up . . . All these works exactly on the sighting line.

Although Watkins never made the connection of these line to energy, in the next year, occultist Dion Fortune published a novel, *The Goat-Foot God*, in which she proposed that leys are "lines of power." Years later, it was suggested that leys follow lines in the cosmic energy of the Earth that can be detected through dowsing.

It is my contention that they are half right. I believe that the leys were created (harnessed and used) by initiates. Think about this: Concentrated thought is powerful stuff. Mind is the builder, as Edgar Cayce said. What if the ancients used their minds to harness the natural energies around and within us and created these lines—to be used over and over—to increase their abilities, to create and build, and to do whatever else they imagined? What if the lines are leftover thought-forms programmed over the years, still playing out their purpose, though no one is left to understand it?

In the book *Ley Lines: Their Nature and Properties: A Dowser's Investigation* (Turnstone Press, 1983), British dowser J. Havelock Fidler wrote that he learned to dowse energy fields with a pendulum and later discovered energy fields were between the stones that make up a ley line. He also discovered that if he hammered a stone, he could "imprint" it with his aura. If he did this with two or more stones, he could create his own ley lines.

Think what you could do if you "imprinted" a circle of stones to be used to circle you while you meditate? Combined with the power of particular scents, you would have a powerful tool.

In a way, prayer is like a thought form. As you attune yourself to the source of all energies, you create a channel of healing, and you send out your healing thought form to transform the one to which it is directed. Other psychic abilities work in much the same way.

When you delve deeper, you find that psychic ability is but one part of soul development. As Cayce said:

Psychic is of the soul. As to whether psychic information is from those who have attuned themselves to the influences that are even in the material world, or to that force or source which has been sent or given in Creative Forces that are constructive in the experience of others, may only be judged by the application of same in the experience of the individual.   5752-5

Keep in mind that, in developing psychic abilities, you are doing so for a purpose. It should be a high purpose, such as furthering your spiritual development or helping others physically or spiritually.

If you have an interest in a particular form of psychic ability, then that probably is where your particular gifts lie. Cayce said there are as many forms of psychic abilities as there are individuals. However, we will deal here with some of the more common.

We will call our efforts experiments. Choose your experiment. You should choose only one on which to work, and it should be the one in which you are most interested. Three times each week, devote an hour to a meditation session, followed by your experiment. You should use the essential oils listed in this chapter, as well as favored scents from previous chapters, to make a blend of scents. You will keep this blend in a closed container and use it for inhalation. After your meditation, inhale your scent, using deep breathing. Breathe in deeply, hold for a moment, exhale. Ten deep breaths should be enough. Then begin the experiment.

To make a blend:

Use the 3-2-1 ratio for the blend to be well balanced. That is, you will have a primary scent with three drops of essential oil, a secondary scent with two drops, and then one drop of a third essential oil as a "bridge" scent. You can, of course, multiply the amounts in this ratio for larger quantities.

Also, a mist of scent can work well here too. To one cup of distilled water, add twenty drops of the first essential oil, ten drops of the second, and five drops of the third. Place this in a spray bottle and shake before use. Before meditation and/or before your psychic experimentation, mist the face, with the eyes closed, or mist the room.

Here's a good blend for the mister:

Sandalwood, 20 drops
Lavender, 10 drops
Rose, 5 drops

CAYCE READINGS ON PSYCHIC ABILITIES

- **Clairvoyance (seeing without the physical eyes)**
- **Clairaudience (hearing without the physical ears)**
- **Clairsentience (sensing feelings through other than the five known senses)**
- **Intuition ("gut" feelings that something is true or false, or right or wrong)**

Trust more and more upon that which may be from within. Or, this is a very common—but a very definite manner to develop:

On any question that arises, ask the mental self—get the answer, yes or no. Rest on that. Do not act immediately (if you would develop the intuitive influences). Then, in meditation or prayer, when looking within self, ask—is this yes or no? The answer is intuitive development. On the same question, to be sure, see? 282-4

Depend more upon the intuitive forces from

within and not harken so much to that of outside influences—but learn to listen to that still small voice from within, remembering as the lesson as was given, not in the storm, the lightning, nor in any of the loud noises as are made to attract man, but rather in the still small voice from within does the impelling influence come to life in an individual that gives for that which must be the basis of human endeavor . . .   239-1

. . . Hence, in governing, in guarding, in guiding such forces, such powers that arise or manifest or demonstrate through the activities of the body, keep the body, the mind, the soul, in attune with the spheres of celestial forces, rather than of earthly forces. Rather than listening to that which is poetically given as to the voice that arises from the earth, listen to that which comes as the music of the spheres . . .   255-12

After meditation, simply ask a question and expect an answer. Also, begin working with the imagination in seeing scenes with the eyes closed. Have a particular reason for doing this. Suppose you want to know whether your employer will be laying off workers. Ask that question in your mind. See whether images appear and whether you can sense an answer. Go with your first impressions. Trust them and give them permission to come through.

- **Psychometry (getting psychic information from objects through touch)**

  (Q) In what way may this be developed and used?
  (A) As given. Application!"   256-2

You can hold something in your hand and get vibrations from it. If an object is owned and loved by someone, it takes on the personality or vibrations of the owner. It's what I call psychic fingerprints. Psychometry is easy if you practice and trust the impressions that come through. Relax, close your eyes while holding the object, and say the first thing that comes into your mind. When doing readings, ask for objects that have been worn a lot or that have special meaning to another. This form of psychic ability is good in helping others locate lost items, lost pets, or children, and in helping solve crimes.

- **Telepathy (mind-to-mind communication)**

    Every entity has clairvoyant, mystic, psychic powers . . .
    First, it must be lived, desired, practised within self, in its dealings with its fellow man. Do not teach that which is only theory. *Live* in thy own experience that thou would teach thy neighbor, thy brother.
    1500-4

    For, as these attune more and more to the awareness of His presence, the desire to know of those influences that may be revealed causes the awareness to become materially practical.
    First, begin between selves. Set a definite time, and each at that moment put down what the other is doing. Do this for twenty days. And ye will find ye have the key to telepathy.   2533-7

Get a partner with whom to experiment. Place two chairs facing one another. Decide who will be the sender and who will be the receiver for this session. Both of you sit in the chairs and hold hands. Close your eyes, and each of you imagine a white beam of energy. Imagine this beam flowing from your hands into the other's, up through the head and through the other's head, down into the arms. It should be like a circle of energy. The sender should think of something (a simple color such as red, blue, green, yellow, or orange; a number from one to ten; or even agree to experiment with choosing red or black). After a few moments, the receiver should give the impression they got. When an answer is given correctly, change roles and let the other send or receive. Later experiments can include names, pictures, etc. And you can even begin to do the experiments with another person who is some distance away. Just be sure to agree on a time and to write down your impressions so you can go back and check them for accuracy.

• Past and Future Lives

In meditation the entity will gain much; not so much as what is ordinarily termed psychic, but rather of the awakening of self's own *experiences* through the many periods in the earth, and the lessons lost or gained there. These, applied in the present experience, especially with that builded in love, will bring the glory of the life well lived, and the blessings from those who contact or know the entity best.   41-71

You can explore past lives with a partner. You also can use a mirror to explore your own past lives alone.

If you are reading another's past life, sit facing one another. Lower the lights in the room so that they are dim and not harsh. Breathe deeply and begin staring into the person's face. Repeat silently that you wish to see a past or future life for that person. After some moments, your partner's facial features will appear to change, and you will see the face as it was in another life or will be in a future life. When you see that face clearly, close your eyes and imagine a scene including that face. It will be the person's past or future life.

To do this for yourself, you will need a mirror set up where you can sit comfortably and go through the same routine. As you stare into the mirror, your face will change. When you see the change clearly, close your eyes, and scenes from that past or future life will manifest.

- **Mediumship (ability to communicate with the spirit world)**

    Also, we will find that, with the attunement of the self in the periods when the body sits for that of the silence, the better *physically* fit the better the *attunement* will be for those active forces of the psychic influences, and of the *connective* rations between the Borderland and the Beyond for the entity; for, as has been given, the voices may be heard by this body when *attuning* self, even as the *vision and* the voice. Keep self attuned. Keep in that way and manner as befitting *that* as is *desired* by the body, for first there is the desire—then there is the proper seeking for that desired. Not as selfish motives, but that self may aid even those *in* the Borderland in their understanding of the relationship of an entity *to* its creative forces, and that which the *soul* seeks. Amen.
    599-8

    As an entity, a soul, a mind, enters—as has been so oft given—put about the self the cloak, the garment, yea the mantle of Christ; not as a man, not as an individual but the *Christ*—that universal consciousness of love that we see manifested in those who have forgotten self but—as Jesus—give themselves that others may know the truth.   1376-1

Cayce advised caution in exercising mediumistic abilities.

The danger was that one might become dependant upon the spirit world and not rely upon self. Here, you must remember that those who have passed on are not all "saints" and that you can come upon "sinners" too. Being in touch with the spirit plane should never be sought for advice, only for solace. Direct communication with loved ones who have passed on can help both the spirit and the one left behind in the physical in that it can demonstrate that life is eternal. Important messages can also be relayed.

After meditation, surround yourself with a prayer of protection. Ask for spirit contact from a specific entity. Wait in expectation. If no response is met after ten minutes, offer a prayer of thanks and, before bedtime, ask again that contact might be made. Cayce said that if there is desire on the part of both parties, contact might be made and that, most often, the contact would come through dreams.

SCENTS FOR PSYCHIC EXPERIMENTS

Fennel
(Foeniculum vulgare)

This has a long history of use as medicine. The early Greek athletes ate the seeds to increase their strength while training for Olympic games. It is associated with longevity and good luck. The scent stimulates the nervous and glandular system. It is balancing, cleansing, purifying, and revitalizing. It has an anise-like scent that has long been believed to offer protection against evil and ward off ill thoughts of others. It is one of nine sacred herbs of the Anglo-Saxons.

Ginger
(Zingiber officinale)

The ancient Greeks and Romans used this in medicines. It comforts, warms, and uplifts while sharpening the senses. It stimulates and grounds and is a powerful nerve tonic. To the natives of Pacific Islands of Dohu, ginger is sacred and used in magic rituals and in medicine. The islanders believe it has a healing effect. It is good in massage and is best when blended with other essential oils.

Hyssop
(Hyssopus officinalis)

This is mentioned in the Bible, and the sweet scent has been used to purify sacred places. It has an ancient reputation as a magical herb. It was one of the bitter herbs used during the Passover ritual. In early times, it was the symbol of baptism and forgiveness of sins. Hebrews and Egyptians used it to sweep out temples. Psalms 51:7, says "Purge me with hyssop and I shall be clean." During pagan rituals, it was sprayed on worshippers to cleanse them. The Greeks used it in similar fashion for the same reason. It was also burned as incense. It uplifts the mind, gives clarity and direction, and calms, while increasing awareness. It is good in massage preparations and as incense.

Caution: Hyssop is not for those with high blood pressure, for children, for pregnant or nursing women, or for the frail.

Immortelle
(Helichrysum angustifolia)

It has a curry-like scent and is valuable as a medicinal plant. It aids detoxification through the lymph glands. It warms and opens and supports deep breathing. It relaxes and elevates the mind. It is thought to increase dream activity or awareness. Good for meditations, imagination, and the creative arts. Use this in massage and for inhalations.

Labdanum
(Cistus ladaniferus)

It was used early as an aromatic and is listed in the Bible as oncha, an ingredient in the ancient temple incense of Moses. It was used by ancient Egyptians as incense and for cosmetic use, and it is abundant on the isles of Crete and Cyprus. It is a resinous oil that gives a characteristic smell to certain glades in Greece. The aromatic material is said to have been sacred to Venus and was burned on altars on the island of Cyprus. It deeply affects the soul and aids mediation, centering, visualization, and spiritual experience, bringing it into the physical. It has a floral scent good for incense and massage.

Neroli
(Citrus aurantium)
This was named for an Italian princess who loved this scent. It is hypnotic, euphoric, and antidepressant. It soothes nerves and relaxes. Today, the white blossoms are used in bridal bouquets as a symbol of purity. It gives a feeling of peace and reenergizes. It is a blood cleanser and helps calm excitability. It is very safe and very relaxing. The blossoms come from the bitter orange tree.

Patchouli
(Pogostemon cablin)
This has a sweet, rich odor that improves with age. It relieves stress and is an important scent in India. Most either love or hate the scent. It stimulates the nervous system and affects the endocrine glands. It is grounding and uplifting. It is sedative in small amounts, stimulating in larger amounts. It increases clarity and balances the endocrine system. Use it in baths or a vaporizer, or in massage.

Rose
(Rosa centifolia)
It was once depicted at a 4,000-year-old palace at Knossos in Crete. It is the first plant matter distilled by Avicenna in his alchemical experiments. It is the symbol of Christian representations of divine love and the symbol used by the Rosicrucian order. St. Domini (1170-1221) was said to have been visited by the Virgin Mary in a mystical vision and received the first rosary made of rose-scented beads. It aids meditation, balances, and calms. It is a mild sedative and antidepressant. In Hindu tradition, it is blended with sandalwood

to form a scent called attar, for ritual use. During the Middle Ages, it was grown in monasteries. It increases concentration.

Thyme
(Thymus vulgaris)
This was one of the first medicinal plants used in the Mediterranean region. It was also used in the embalming rituals in ancient Egypt. It was offered to Venus and other gods as incense. The Romans bathed in waters scented with thyme for courage. It is good for depression and is relaxing and cleansing. It energizes on the emotional, mental, and physical levels. It is said to be a tonic. It has a mystical connection in that it is believed to be able to let one see fairies (or the other world), and so it is a bridge to another dimension.

Ylang Ylang
(Cananga odorata)
This scent is calming and soothing. It is euphoric and narcotic. It has a calming effect on the heart chakra. It regulates the adrenaline. It relaxes the central nervous system and is good for panic, anger, and stress. It is an intoxicating scent, good against depression and apathy. It sedates and regulates the heart on a physical and emotional level. It is a heady, floral scent.

CAYCE READINGS ON PSYCHIC DEVELOPMENT,

Psychic means of the *spirit* or *soul,* for cooperation of the Phenomena, or manifestation of the workings of those forces within the individual, or through the individual, from whom such phenomena, or of such phases of the working of the spirit and soul, to bring the actions of these to the physical plane . . .

Psychic in the broader sense meaning spirit, soul, or the imagination of the mind, when attuned to the various phases of either of these two portions of the entity of an individual, or from the entity of others who are passed into the other planes than the physical or material; yet in the broader sense, the Phenomena of Psychic forces are as material as the forces that become visible to the material or physical plane.

3744-1

As there developed more of the individual association with material conditions, and they partook of same in such a manner as to become wholly or in part a portion *of* same, farther—or more hidden, more unseen—has become occult or psychic manifestations. First there were the occasional harking back. Later by dream. Again we find individuals raised in certain sections for specific purposes. As the cycle has gone about, time and again has there arisen in the earth those that *manifested* these forces in a more magnificent, more beneficent, way and manner.   364-11

Psychic is of the soul; the abilities to reason *by* the faculties or by the mind of the soul. And when this is done, enter into the inner self, opening self through the ideals of the meditation that have been presented through these channels, and surrounding self with the consciousness of the Christ that He may guide in that as will be shown thee; either in writing (inspirationally, not hand guided) or in the intuitive forces that come from the deeper meditation, may there come much that would guide self first. Do not seek first the material things, but rather spiritual guidance, developing self to the attunement to the psychic forces of the spheres as through the experiences in the varied activities in the varied planes of experience, but ever in the light of that promise that has been given to be known among men, "If ye love me, keep my commandments, that I may come and abide with thee and bring to thy remembrance those things that thou has need of that have been *between* me and thee since the foundations of the world!   513-1

First—as was indicated to these of old—purge or purify thy body—whether this be by mental means or by ablutions, do it in that manner as to satisfy thine own conscience.

Then enter into the holy of holies of thine own inner self; for there He hat promised to meet thee. Let thy prayer be as this:

As I surround myself with the consciousness of the Christ-Mind, may I—in body, in purpose, in desire—be purified to become the channel through which He may *direct* me in that *He,* the Christ, would have me do;" as respecting an individual, a condition, an experience. And as ye wait on Him, the answer will come.   1947-3

(Q) What is the highest possible psychic realization . . . ?

(A) That God, the Father, speaks directly to the sons of men—even as He has promised.   440-4

Bibliography

Bible, The King James Version. World Publishing Co. New York, N.Y. 1971.

Budge, E.A. Wallis. *The Book of the Dead.* Gramercy Books, Avenel, N.Y. 1995

Devereux, Paul. *Shamanism and the Mystery Lines.* Llewellyn, St. Paul, Minn. 1994.

Frazer, Sir James. *The New Golden Bough* (Rev. and ed. by Theodor H. Gaster) Criterion Books, New York, N.Y. 1964.

Gibson, Walter B., and Litzka R. *The Complete Illustrated Book of the Psychic Sciences.* Simon & Schuster, New York, N.Y. 1976.

Hitching, Francis. *Earth Magic.* Simon & Schuster, New York, N.Y. 1976.

LaBerge, Stephen, and Rhingold, Howard. *Exploring the World of Lucid Dreaming.* Ballantine Books, New York, N.Y. 1987.

Mystic Places. Time-Life Books, Time Warner Bookmarks. 1970.

Pohle, Nancy C., and Selover, Ellen L. *Awakening the Real You: Awareness Through Dreams and Intuition* A.R.E. Press, Virginia Beach, Va. 1999.

Stewart, Louis. *Life Forces: A Contemporary Guide to the Cult and Occult* Universal Press Syndicate, New York, N.Y. 1980.

Tisserand, Robert. Interview: "In Profile: John Steele." *The International Journal of Aromatherapy*, Vol. 5, No. 1, Spring 1993.

Van Auken, John. *The End Times.* A.R.E. Press, Virginia Beach, Va.

Van Auken, John. "Success With Meditation", Reflections: A Commentary on the Edgar Cayce Readings," Vol. 1, No. 2, August 1992, Edgar Cayce Foundation.

Index

O

Oak 29
OBE 67, 68, 71, 73
Obsession(s) 20, 113
Olfactory 35, 36, 38, 39, 42, 45, 46
Olive oil 72, 114
Oncha 129
Oracle(s) 32
Orange 46, 85, 88, 125, 130
Orris root 39, 42, 43
Out-of-body experience/travel—also
    see OBE 64, 67, 68

P

Parathyroid 91
Patchouli 130
Peach blossom 44
Peanut oil 114
Pelvic bone 85, 88
Pepper(s) 46, 48
Perfume 20, 25, 26, 32, 35, 40, 41, 44,
    81, 82
Peyote 30
Pine 28
Pineal gland 68
Pituitary 16, 91
Plant(s) ix, 6, 8, 21, 23, 26, 28, 30, 32,
    37, 40, 46, 61, 69, 82, 113, 118, 129,
    130, 131
Poison(s)/-ous 46, 82
Potassium nitrate 78
Potpourri 4, 79
Powder(s) 77, 78
Prayer 97
Prayer/pray 27, 30, 75, 93, 96, 97, 102,
    105, 106, 107, 108, 109, 111, 115,
    120, 122, 127, 133
Precognition 17, 57, 68
Pregnant/pregnancy ix, 79, 129
Priest(s) 8, 13, 17, 26, 27, 30, 32, 34
Prophecy/prophetic 17, 32, 68
Pshchic 126
Psychic 2, 3, 4, 12, 17, 23, 34, 40, 41, 49,
    50, 51, 55, 56, 57, 60, 61, 62, 67,
    68, 69, 70, 71, 75, 76, 77, 86, 88,
    89, 90, 96, 104, 116, 118, 120, 121,
    122, 123, 124, 125, 128, 131, 132,
    133
Psychometry 77, 123, 124
Purification 24, 27, 31, 80, 112, 113

Q

Quartz 8, 19

R

Raisins 78
Red 85, 88, 125
Reincarnation 8, 16
Research 3, 5, 7, 8, 11, 21, 22, 23, 24, 29,
    34, 35, 36, 37, 38, 44, 65, 68, 105
Resin(s) 21, 23, 25, 77, 80, 81, 111, 129
Retrocognition 17
Rose 17, 32, 36, 41, 45, 83, 112, 113, 122,
    130
Rosemary 37, 82

S

Sage 30, 66, 72
Salt 78, 112
Saltpeter 78
Sand 59, 78
Sandalwood 26, 30, 31, 39, 43, 44, 47,
    78, 82, 113, 122, 130
Sarcophagus 45
Scent(s) ix, 4, 19, 20, 22, 23, 24, 28, 30,
    31, 33, 34, 35, 36, 37, 38, 40, 41,
    43, 57, 61, 66, 70, 72, 78, 79, 80,
    81, 82, 83, 84, 111, 112, 113, 121,
    128, 129, 130, 131
Sedative 35, 69, 70, 81, 83, 100, 130
Seed(s) 7, 23, 41, 82, 110, 128
Self-confidence 89
Sempervirens 111
Serotonin 35
Sexual energy 24
Sexuality/sex/sexual 36, 88
Shaman(s)/-ism 3, 13, 30, 135
Silver cord 73
Sin(s) 47, 113, 117
Skin 14, 22, 23, 37
Sleep 28, 36, 55, 57, 61, 62, 63, 64, 65,
    66, 69, 70, 71, 72, 73, 113
Smell(s) 20, 23, 27, 36, 37, 38, 39, 40,
    42, 45, 49, 129
Smoke 21, 25, 26, 31, 32, 75, 77, 78, 81,
    112
Smudging 30
Snake(s)/serpent(s) 5, 9, 10, 11, 13, 14,
    16
Soma 91